COPING SUCCESSFULLY WITH PAIN

NEVILLE SHONE was a university lecturer and a keen sportsman with a busy social life until a spinal disease rendered him almost immobile and in constant pain, forcing him out of work and bringing him close to despair. *Coping Successfully With Pain* describes the techniques of pain management which enabled him to regain his mobility and his zest for life, and to escape from the prison of pain. Neville is also the author of *Cancer – A Family Affair* (Sheldon Press, 1995).

Overcoming Common Problems Series

For a full list of titles please contact
Sheldon Press, Marylebone Road, London NW1 4DU

Overcoming Common Problems Series

Overcoming Common Problems Series

Overcoming Common Problems

COPING SUCCESSFULLY WITH PAIN

Neville Shone

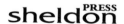
sheldon PRESS

First published in Great Britain 1992
Sheldon Press, SPCK, Marylebone Road, London NW1 4DU

Revised and updated edition 1995
Fourth impression 2001

Illustrations by Cheryl Quinn

British Library Cataloguing-in-Publication Data

A catalogue record for this book is available from the British Library

ISBN 0–85969–750–9

Photoset by Deltatype Ltd, Ellesmere Port, Cheshire
Printed in Great Britain by Biddles Ltd
www.biddles.co.uk

A journey of a thousand miles must begin
. . . with a single step

Lao-tze 550 BC

Contents

Acknowledgements

Thanks are due for the continued help and support of:

Dr Christopher Wells, Consultant in Pain Relief and Director of Pain Management Programme, and

Dr Eric Ghadiali, Consultant Clinical Psychologist, both of the Walton Centre for Neurology and Neurosurgery, Liverpool.

The late Helen Yaffe-Smith, Spiritual Healer, who for many years contributed to the work of the Pain Management Programme at Walton and who provided me personally with a great deal of encouragement.

Jim Tapper, formerly a member of the team at Walton and now Principal Clinical Psychologist, Southport and Formby Health Authority.

John Ball, who has not only provided support but has allowed me to use his story in Chapter 6 for the benefit of others.

Prof. Wilbert Fordyce of the University of Washington Hospital, Seattle, whose research and clinical practice have done much to further the multi-disciplinary approach to the treatment of pain throughout the world. He has generously provided me with original research material and continued over the years to provide me with personal support in my own work in bringing the pain management message to the general public.

Prof. Terry Murphy and the Staff of the Pain Management Programme, University of Washington Hospital, Seattle, who allowed me to participate fully with them in their work with people in pain.

Pain Association Scotland who, under their former name of PLUS, developed a network of self-help support groups for people with pain and cancer throughout Scotland. They have carried on their work quietly and effectively for many years. I am sorry it took me so long to become aware of their work but I am grateful for their initiative in inviting me to develop my ideas about bringing the pain management approach into the community and for encouraging me to put the ideas of this book into practice.

Those Members and Staff of Pain Association Scotland who participated in the introductory community-based self-help training programme for group leaders and individual pain sufferers, held in Glasgow during the autumn of 1994. Many of the ideas in the final chapter have been refined as a result of this original venture.

Cheryl Quinn whose instructive illustrations have brightened the text.

Thanks are due, not least, for the fellowship of all those brave people who are learning how to enjoy life again in spite of their pain, including the many people who took the trouble to contact me after reading the first edition of this book. I continue to learn a lot from all of them.

And, finally, Sheldon Press for their constant encouragement and for giving me the opportunity to produce this second edition.

Neville Shone
Arbroath
May 1995

Introduction

If you or someone close to you has had a pain problem for more than three months then this book is for you. If a book such as this had been available to me some years ago then I may not have wasted so much time sinking into disability whilst waiting for the 'magical cure'. It is a practical guide to handling the many situations that you once dealt with automatically but which now may seem daunting, and hopefully, will eliminate some of the fears which may confront you.

It may be that you find it difficult to stand or sit for very long, or walk more than a few yards or feel so miserable as a result of your pain that life has lost its savour. Sitting, standing and walking are crucial to functioning and our inability to do them comfortably limits our scope to such an extent that we tend to avoid getting involved and as a result miss out on the rich variety that life has to offer.

My aim, therefore, is to help you understand the nature of the problem and to put you in a better position to ask informed questions of professionals involved in your treatment, and, in addition, to provide a pointer to the steps which you can take in planning and carrying out your own treatment and rehabilitation in a way that meets your own individual needs. Keep it by you for reference and use it as a handbook.

I am not suggesting that you disregard the advice of your doctors; I simply wish to provide you with a set of positive options which you can use to become less dependent on external sources and to find the confidence to rely more on your own resources in managing your pain. At this point you may be tempted to say, 'Ah!, but nobody understands my pain like I do.' Maybe not, but I have had to learn to understand and deal with my own pain and resulting disability over many years and to communicate this understanding to others whose lives, like mine, have been shattered by the experience. However, first-hand experience, although valuable, is not enough. We need to have access to knowledge and information about the problem itself, the techniques and skills required to deal

1

with it, and where and how these can be acquired. In developing my understanding of the problem and methods of working, I have drawn upon my knowledge and experience of pain from both sides of the fence as patient and therapist and from my professional training and experience working with children and families.

My own pain problem, which is the result of a spinal disease, began in the mid-1970s and I became progressively incapacitated so that by the end of 1981 I was no longer able to work as a university teacher and as a result had to take premature retirement. My social life had become severely restricted and I had changed from being an outgoing energetic sportsman and keen amateur stage performer to spending my days confined to the house, afraid to move even slightly for fear of injury. The pain made it difficult to get off to sleep at night and when eventually I did, it woke me again. It was a chore to get out of bed in the morning and I spent the day feeling only half awake. The pain was on my mind almost constantly.

My condition caused confusion to friends and family since there were no outward signs of illness apart from the fact that my face was gaunt and grey. But I could no longer sit for more than a few minutes at a time or hold a book comfortably; even when the book was supported, I was unable to concentrate for more than a few minutes. As an academic whose professional life was dependent on extensive reading this was devastating: comparable to a craftsman losing the use of his hand. I shuffled about like an out-of-condition octogenarian. I was 44 years old! As far as I was concerned I was locked in the prison of pain until the day I died or until someone came along with the key, in the form of a cure, to set me free. I was full of despair and afraid. Afraid particularly that I would become mentally unbalanced, frightened that I would never, ever be in a position to thoroughly enjoy myself again or to join in everyday activities such as going out for a meal, country walks, or sitting in the theatre. In short, the future looked bleak and this is the way things remained until. . . .

In the spring of 1985 I was offered a place on the Pain Management Programme run by Walton Hospital in Liverpool under the directorship of Dr Christopher Wells. No 'quick fix' was promised. The only offer made to me on entering the programme was that at the end of four weeks' daily attendance I would be more mobile and better able to cope with my pain. Dr Wells was the first doctor to focus on my pain as the real problem. Hitherto the emphasis had been on investigation, possible treatment – and cure, a process which seemed to have gone on endlessly. As I had long since lost interest in the cause of the pain and was desperate for some relief, his words were music to my ears. Although modest objectives were claimed for the programme, I and many others found that surprising, unexpected and wonderful things can happen as a result of taking this step. The programme, which had been running for about a year, was staffed by a dedicated group of people, medical and non-medical, who firmly believed in its aims and accepted above all that PAIN . . . IS . . . REAL. Although similar programmes exist in the United States, this was the first of its kind in Europe. In contrast to its American counterparts, like so many pioneer ventures in this country, it was given official approval and encouragement but relied for the most part on grants and fund-raising efforts and the unpaid services of many of the staff.

As a result of this programme I regained my zest for life and learned many skills fundamental to building up strength, resuming mobility and controlling my pain. My progress was helped by the fact that at the end of the four-week course I was invited to make a voluntary contribution to the programme as a therapist. Before I could undertake this I had to be sure that I was physically able to cope with driving once or twice a week from North Wales to Liverpool and at the end of the journey still have sufficient energy to work to good effect for two hours at a time with a group of 8–12 patients, and then drive home again! This tested out the effectiveness of the teaching of Dr Wells and his colleagues and although at first I needed several days to recover between each trip, I found in a matter of weeks that it was well within my capacity and I began to set new targets for myself. Ultimately, I set myself the target of writing a book which would help people in circumstances similar to my own and to demonstrate how available resources can be used much more effectively in the treatment of chronic pain.

It has taken me about seven years to build up sufficient stamina to enable me to carry out research, both in this country and in America, and to meld experience, practice and information into book form. Nothing is recommended which I have not tried myself. I still cope with pain every day and feel that I can offer a great deal to others who are just getting to grips with managing their pain or who have been locked into pain for many years without having had the opportunity to learn effective ways of coping.

Like the pain management programme, which I shall cover more fully in a later chapter, this book will help you, step by step, to draw on all available resources, external and internal, to regain control over your pain and your own life. You can do this provided you accept that your problem has taken time to develop, that it has been with you a long time, and that it will take time to sort out. So, what is my aim? In fact, I have several:

1. To help you understand your pain and make the best use of the professional help which is available;
2. To help you by physical and psychological means to find ways of controlling your body's alarm system which is causing you so much discomfort;
3. To help you increase your range of physical mobility and activity;
4. To help you understand the connection between your pain, your feelings, and your behaviour, and how they all interact, and to demonstrate how you can change them for the better and help you to enjoy a fuller life.

Ultimately, the test of the programme is that you will behave differently and feel better.

The basic premise on which this programme is built is that you have inside you the resources to promote your own healing and that you have the will to get better. You will not be able to achieve this single-handed. You need to be shown the way. You need to be shown the way to recognize and strengthen your own resources and progressively to learn new ways of thinking, feeling and behaving. By following this step-by-step guide you will be able to look back and see that what was once thought to be insurmountable has been conquered and you are already well on your way to meeting a new challenge.

1

Understanding Chronic Pain

The extent of the problem

It is estimated that 11% of the adult population of Britain suffers from long lasting or chronic pain. As you might expect, the numbers increase with age so that 22% of people over the age of 65 suffer from this type of pain.

Chronic pain is no respecter of youth. There is considerable evidence from attendance figures at pain clinics that children and teenagers are also affected. As you can imagine, young people who suffer in this way must find it very traumatic to have their physical, emotional and social development so seriously threatened.

Chronic pain defined

You may be familiar with the colloquial misuse of the word 'chronic' and have heard the expression 'It hurts something chronic!' meaning, 'The pain is severe'. In fact 'chronic' is derived from the Greek word for time and relates to pain which is persistent and generally constant rather than intermittent. It may be severe at times but at other times it may be dull and at a level which is enough to remind you of its presence, gnawing away at your stamina. Like a chronic illness, it may be long-standing and last for months or years rather than days or weeks.

Problems which give rise to short bursts of pain, perhaps on a weekly or monthly basis include such things as migraine, tension headaches, forms of neuralgia and pre-menstrual pain. Quite often the pain, although severe, will last just a few hours or days, leaving the person to carry on normally for the rest of the time. This kind of pain may be referred to as 'chronic periodic pain' and often responds to simple treatments. Because of its chronic nature it may begin to dominate the way a person lives, feels, thinks and behaves, and limit enjoyment of life in just the same way as chronic pain itself.

It is generally accepted that, initially, pain is a signal that the body is under attack – cuts, broken bones, knocks, or an internal injury or disease process. It is an alarm that calls for attention. If the cause of the pain is treated appropriately then it usually goes away. It is short-lived, lasting perhaps no more than six months at the outside. Pain of this nature is usually referred to as 'acute' pain and is regarded as 'useful' pain. This is in contrast to pain which arrives too late to warn us, for example cancer pain which may come long after the disease process is established, and as such may be regarded as 'useless' pain.

Chronic pain may also be regarded as 'useless' pain because it continues – sometimes in the absence of any illness or injury or long after healing has taken place and the pain has served its purpose. Nevertheless, the pain is REAL and it is long lasting.

Some conditions giving rise to chronic pain

The strange and possibly meaningless language used by the computer industry is a mystery to most of us. If you are a gardener you will know that plants are given Latin names to convey to gardeners throughout the world a whole host of information. The medical profession, too, use terms which are helpful to the professionals when they communicate with each other. A term like 'Sciatica' conveys to a medical practitioner in one word a whole lot of information about a specific illness which could take several pages of descriptive information to do the same thing. You can appreciate that it is very useful to be able to do this. However, when the layman hears technical words used to describe illnesses they can sound strange and even frightening, particularly if you know of other people, perhaps in your own family, who have possibly developed extreme forms of these illnesses. The process of labelling, whilst making it easy for the professionals to communicate with each other can, in fact, create a barrier between the professionals and the patients they serve. Your illness may have been labelled. You may have been told you are suffering from some form of arthritic or rheumatic condition. If this is the case then it may have been given a more specific label such as osteoarthritis, rheumatoid arthritis, osteoporosis, spondylitis, curvature of the spine, spinal stenosis, sciatica, facet joint pain or, perhaps, erythema nodosum. These are just some of the words used by doctors to convey information about the specific rheumatic and arthritic illnesses. There are probably many more. These illnesses are well described and there are various clinical tests which indicate their presence. Each one of them, under certain conditions, can lead to chronic pain.

There are other problems relating to the spine and central nervous system which are notorious producers of chronic pain. Things like ruptured or bulging lumbar or cervical discs causing severe back, neck and head pain which may radiate down the legs or the arms. There is a whole group of illnesses which go under the label 'neuralgia': for example, trigeminal neuralgia, post-herpetic neuralgia (pain after Shingles). Post-operative adhesions, scar tissue, tissue damage, and nerve irritation caused by tumours can all lead to prolonged and persistent pain.

There are other pains which are not so easily explained and extensive tests and investigations may not always reveal a specific cause. For example, migraine, causalgia and residual pain following injury long after healing has taken place, phantom limb pain where real pain exists where the amputated limb once was, repeated unaccountable muscle spasm, low back pain, recurring headaches, neck and shoulder pain.

Then there is the pain which results from standing or sitting badly, or working in positions where exceptional strain is persistently applied to one part, or one side of the body. Problems arising in this way may take a long time to develop but unless recognized and corrected can lead to chronic conditions. Candidates for this type of problem are supermarket check-out staff who continually handle goods to the left side whilst keying in prices or codes with their right hand, or the typist who has a badly adjusted chair. Then again, muscles can be put under too much tension by using more effort than is necessary when carrying out everyday tasks. As a result, muscle spasms may occur causing soft tissue damage and unless the cause is remedied, the pain will persist. The amount of tension in muscles when being used can be measured and it may be necessary to teach ways of using muscles more efficiently. Unless such help is given it is possible that pain arising from this cause will persist.

Paradoxically, medication prescribed or bought over the counter to obtain symptomatic relief may in fact precipitate a pain problem.

Unfortunately there is a tendency for medication to be misused by medical practitioners and patients alike. It is too easy to slip into the habit of giving and receiving repeat prescriptions, increasing dosages, mixing incompatible substances and mixing drugs with alcohol. Herbal and homeopathic remedies fall into the same category and it is wrong to think that you cannot overdose on 'natural' remedies.

We usually think of pain as a physical problem but it can be triggered and sustained by emotional factors. Fears, anxieties and conflicts may produce tension, muscle spasm, tightness in chest muscles, low back pain, head and neck pain; and people going through emotional difficulties can find that they feel weak, sick, cold and they may even have difficulty walking.

You are probably familiar with the expression 'I was deeply hurt', or 'I was deeply wounded', signifying that someone has had an experience which has left them feeling as if they have been physically attacked. This can happen as a result of losing a job, losing a partner, having unkind things said about you, being let down by someone you trust or being the victim of a crime or even an unwelcome sexual overture. Such experiences can produce a long-lasting feeling of dis-ease within the person who may not even relate the discomfort to the bad experience but the feelings of discomfort may persist long after the incident which caused the hurt has been forgotten and may culminate in a chronic pain condition.

Sometimes the term 'psychogenic pain' is used to describe chronic pain which has no apparent physical cause. Research shows that in older people particularly, pain can be a disguised form of depression. It has also been found that people who have phobias, particularly about going out, can develop pain whilst remaining unaware that they have the phobia. In a small number of cases, chronic pain offers an acceptable way of avoiding something unpleasant such as a disagreeable occupation, a demanding partner or a stressful family situation. People who suffer in this way are certainly not to be branded as work-shy or weak in any way. They feel just as distressed about their condition as anyone else and often they are not consciously aware of the complicated psychological mechanism giving rise to the condition.

Pain is not always a physical experience

It may be that you have picked up this book because you feel somehow that you hurt inside even though you may not have a physical pain or symptom. Many of us have difficulty coming to terms with normal experiences such as loss and separation and may be weighed down by emotional burdens. You may feel that your problem is too trivial to merit the attention of your doctor or other professional helpers even though it is handicapping and limits your ability to enjoy life. Although this is outside the accepted definition of chronic pain nevertheless I think it is important to acknowledge this aspect of suffering and treat it as another form of pain. If you recognize that this applies to you, then you may find in this book the means of regaining control and lost vitality.

It is my belief that any problem, whether it manifests itself physically or emotionally, affects the whole person. It is the whole person therefore who needs treatment. This book is about treating the whole person irrespective of the label which has been attached to the problem.

Whatever the label, whatever the cause, the common denominator is . . . PAIN!

Untangling the web

In recent years ideas about pain have changed considerably. It was once thought that pain was a straightforward relationship between the body and the brain. It was assumed that anything which happened to injure the body internally or externally triggered off a signal which was conveyed directly via the nerves to the brain. It was believed that the intensity of the pain was proportional to the degree of damage and that if injury or damage could not be detected, then pain could not really exist. Where no obvious physical condition could be found to account for the pain it was often assumed that patients complaining of pain were malingering. It is now known that pain is a much more complex phenomenon and anybody working in the treatment of pain must take into account not only knowledge about its physiology but also understand the variety of ways in which people respond to it in different situations. They must also be aware of the complex feelings and attitudes surrounding pain and understand the influence of family life, the kind of work the patient does, the duration of the problem and the effects of earlier medical treatment.

This understanding is basic to professionals working in the field but you, too, must be able to assess for yourself the many and sometimes interwoven factors which are operating in and around you. This book will try to bring you this understanding which you can use in taking responsibility for directing your own recovery. Remember, knowledge is power!

In order to provide a basis for your understanding I should like at this stage to outline some of the current thinking about pain. It is inevitable that some technical references will be made in order to avoid the risk of over-simplification but I hope this will not deter you from reading on and gaining more understanding about the reasons for some of the treatment ideas proposed later in the book.

Pain and the different ways in which people respond to it

Although pain is a physical sensation, the amount of pain we feel depends very much on the situation in which we experience it. We can even choose to ignore it, consciously or unconsciously. As a child you probably played out on a bitterly cold day and got thoroughly involved in a snowball fight. Your gloves got in the way of good snowball-making so you took them off, ignoring the agony of the icy cold of the snowball in your hands. Not until your mother dragged you indoors wet and bedraggled did you realize just how cold and painful your fingers were. You will agree, therefore, that there is more to pain than mere sensation.

We are all familiar with heroic tales of soldiers injured in battle fighting on regardless and only being aware of their pain once the battle ended. Research carried out in the 1950s showed that soldiers with severe wounds complained less about their pain and required less medication than did civilians facing an operation. Those facing surgery were anxious about the idea of being in hospital, being separated from their family, and about the outcome of the operation, whereas soldiers who had severe wounds faced the positive outcome of being removed from the conflict to safety in hospital and a likely return home. It must be concluded, therefore, that the individual's experience of pain relates to the situation in which it arises.

You may have found that when you are busy and totally involved in an interesting task you can forget the pain altogether. You may also have noticed that certain activities can be enjoyed in comparative comfort whilst at other times the pain increases. Shopping for food may bring on the pain whereas going to buy a new outfit may be quite pleasurable. Just take note of those things that lessen your pain and those which increase it.

The way in which the brain perceives pain and how it sets about combating it

With a few exceptions (for example, those suffering from leprosy) most of us are equipped with nerve-endings throughout the body which detect potentially dangerous physical stimuli – e.g. cuts, burns, knocks. These particular nerve-endings are referred to as 'pain receptors'. The pain message received at these points is conveyed via bunches of nerve fibres to other nerve fibres and hence to cells in the spinal cord for direct transmission to the brain. This route or pathway is called the Ascending Tract.

Research has shown that pain is not always conveyed along a single route. It can be transmitted at super-fast speed along one pathway or slowly and continuously along another. This is because the nerve fibres which transmit the pain messages are of different size and at different depths from the surface of the body. It might be helpful to imagine a road network with motorways transmitting the pain very quickly and a number of minor roads transmitting the pain rather more slowly. Large-diameter A-beta nerve fibres are the motorways and the smaller-diameter A-delta and C nerve fibres are the minor roads. It is the slow C-fibre pain which is often associated with chronic problems.

In addition to these nerve fibres conveying the pain messages at different speeds, there are variations in the quality of pain along the different routes. Very simply, it is helpful to think about fast pain as being the kind of pain which conveys the message that an impact has taken place, in other words, the feeling of pressure and touch. The A-delta pain (one of the slow routes) may be experienced as sharp or stabbing, and the C-fibre pain may be experienced as a dull aching sensation.

The spinal cord is the main route for conveying all pain messages to and from the brain and it is in the spinal cord that the pain message gets switched either to the fast or the slow route.

Just as there is a route which conveys the pain to the brain, there is another route, usually called the Descending Tract, down which the brain attempts to counteract the pain messages which are trying to make their way up. Along this downward pathway the brain transmits messages for chemical substances to be released so that 'gates' in the spinal cord can be closed to block off ascending messages. These chemical substances are usually referred to as neurotransmitters and act as painkillers. They can also act as pain producers when called upon to sound the alarm of illness or injury.

The body is quite capable of producing its own natural painkillers and a group of neurotransmitters (endorphins and enkephalins) has been identified which can have the same effect as morphine or heroin. People produce differing amounts of these natural pain-killers and therefore show different capacities to close the gate to the pain messages and hence experience more or less pain than others.

The way in which we can assist in this process

It has been demonstrated that in certain circumstances the body can be helped to produce more or less of these neurotransmitters. The production of these positive neurotransmitters is helped by exercise, relaxation, positive thinking and enjoyable activity. It is said that it is these chemicals which help to produce the joggers' 'high' or that special serene feeling which occurs after lovemaking.

At this stage we can expand a little more on the idea of the 'gate'. It is common practice for mothers instinctively to rub a pain away or 'kiss it better' when a child hurts itself. These actions effectively close the gate to the pain being experienced. But why are they so effective?

In 1965 Doctors Melzack and Wall suggested the idea of 'gates' existing on the nerve-fibres in the spinal cord that can either open to allow pain impulses through to the brain, or close to cut them off. The Gate-Control Theory (as it is known) proposes that a sufficient amount of stimuli can close the gates to the pain sensation. Hence, the rubbing of an injury produces a sensation which is conveyed to the brain at a faster speed along the motorway (the large-diameter nerve fibres) and in effect close the gate to the messages being carried along the minor roads (the small-diameter nerve fibres). This is a similar reaction to that produced by the chemical messages from the brain instructing the gates to close on the pain sensation.

Some of the factors which inhibit our ability to cope with pain

Prolonged inactivity, drug dependency, and negative feelings have been shown to suppress the production of endorphins and enkephalins thus reducing a person's capacity to cope with pain.

Perhaps it would be easier to find a way of dealing with pain if its base were purely physiological – but we know it is not. It is much more complex than that. It is very difficult to distinguish the sensation of pain from the suffering it causes. The severity of the pain is very often measured by the amount of suffering the patient feels. Suffering relates not only to the pain sensation itself but to the individual's feelings, thoughts, and behaviour which result from the pain. It is these subjective elements which prolong and possibly increase the pain.

There is a very close relationship between the mind and the body. This relationship must be understood if we are to begin to understand and treat the problem of chronic pain. Good examples of this relationship are found in situations which cause nervousness or anxiety; perhaps anticipating an examination, a visit to the dentist or hospital, or waiting your turn to appear on stage, and you will remember the butterflies in the tummy, the tight dry mouth and throat, and perhaps an urge to go to the toilet. These anxieties relate to memories of previous experiences or fear of the unknown. In a similar way you may have vivid memories of pain from the past and these memories in themselves may produce anxiety and tension which can magnify your present experience of pain.

This complex psychological mechanism becomes even more powerful when you think that we have the capacity to imagine and anticipate the future. Anticipation and imagination can provoke the thought: 'If the pain is bad now and I am losing my ability to do all the things I enjoy, what is it going to be like in the next few weeks, months, or even years?' This, in turn, will prompt even more anxiety and tension to exacerbate the present pain. Talking about pain, dwelling on it, and on other peoples' problems, will only reinforce your pain sensation. As you talk about your pain and remember occasions when things have been difficult, you trigger off memories which can actually bring about physiological changes which make the pain real.

Testing the theories

Now, test out some of the processes I have described for yourself. First read through this paragraph and then close your eyes and think about an occasion which you found very enjoyable, perhaps a day by the sea. Feel the warmth of the sun on your back. Remember the sound of the waves, the children on the beach, sniff that special smell of the sea. Fill out the scene in your mind's eye. See the colour of the sky reflected in the water, the sun sparkling on the tops of the waves. Relive the experience. Enjoy it fully. You can rest now and enjoy that feeling for as long as you wish, and on this occasion it hasn't cost you anything! Take account of the way you feel, the degree of comfort, and your level of relaxation.

If you are not entirely convinced of this relationship between the mind and body, try another little exercise. Sit in your chair and imagine that you are in a train on your way to London – certain that at the end of the journey you are going to receive bad news about someone close to you. Stay in this position for a minute or two and then come out of the experience completely.

Now, imagine that you are in a train on your way to London knowing that at the end of the journey you will be presented with a cheque for a million pounds which you have won on the pools!

Now compare the way you sat, the way you felt on each occasion. Be aware of the differences in your behaviour, noting the change in facial expression, your posture, the tension in the muscles of your hands, your shoulders, neck and stomach.

Long-standing pain produces exhaustion and limits the capacity to cope with everyday activities which were previously carried out without effort. This fall-off in capacity produces feelings of inadequacy, lowered self-esteem, anger, anxiety, fear, frustration and an overriding feeling that everything is out of control. The result is deep sadness and even depression.

The pain and the feelings may not appear obvious to the onlooker but the person experiencing pain may consciously, or unconsciously, signal the extent of the suffering in a number of ways. Deep gasps and sighs, holding painful parts of the body, walking and moving awkwardly, outbursts of impatience, tearfulness, general grouchiness, long periods of silence, retiring to bed and withdrawing from company generally. This suffering disturbs family, social, and work relationships. These disturbances in their turn increase the feelings of inadequacy, lowered self-esteem, anger, frustration, depression and add *guilt* to the long list. This feeling of guilt may not only belong to the sufferer but also to everyone else around who feel too inadequate to help. Suffering, then, becomes the universal experience, the common bond, the link which holds – or divides – the family and close friends.

The strategy for treatment

Until recently, treatment for chronic pain has been based on the assumption that if there is pain, there must be an underlying cause which must be found and corrected before the pain and its associated problems can be relieved. This view is useful when dealing with the onset of any new pain but as time passes and the pain becomes chronic, a different level of understanding is required. Any strategy for treating chronic pain must address the whole problem of the pain, the suffering, and the accompanying behaviour. This is a tall order especially when your pain appears to be an insurmountable obstacle. This book lays out the strategy which addresses the total problem and you will find that your pain is not such an insurmountable obstacle as you think.

In the following pages I will tell you the story of Karen. . . .

2
The Way In

By definition, chronic pain does not happen overnight. By the time your condition is recognized as chronic pain, no matter what its cause, you will have gone through exhaustive medical tests, examinations and diagnostic interviews. You may have been on medication for months, or even years, had physiotherapy or surgery. You may even have sought advice or treatment from various complementary medical practitioners and by now have reached the point where you are thoroughly fed up with the whole business. You may have lost faith in the ability of the professionals to help you and feel that no one understands you or your problem. Your sense of isolation and helplessness is wearing you down and adding to your problems. To find out how this state of affairs can come about, let us take a closer look at a specific case.

As you read Karen's story, try to spot those factors which have contributed to the build up of her chronic pain state. Doing this will enable you to get a clearer perspective on the way the chronic pain state is reached. At the end I will highlight some points for you to compare with your own interpretation and comment on them in the light of present thinking.

Karen and her husband Ken are in their late thirties. They have two children in their early teens. When she was 33 Karen developed severe back pain after moving heavy furniture. Her doctor advised complete bed rest, pain-killers and muscle relaxants.

This was the first time Karen had been off work since the children started school. At first Karen quite enjoyed the rest but when after a week the pain was no better, she became concerned and not a little frustrated. She had two main concerns, the extra workload on the family, and her job. She was a retail merchandiser, driving around the Northwest of England and the Borders delivering goods to customers and arranging shop displays.

Karen rested for another week, just getting up in the evenings or to make herself the odd cup of tea. Ken coped with the evening meal, drove the children to school, did the shopping and cleaning, on top of his own job. Karen was by now finding it difficult to straighten up and was feeling weak. This increased her anxiety.

She was unable to give a firm date to her employers about returning to work and was unhappy that they were already talking about making alternative arrangements to look after their customers.

Her doctor advised her not to worry but to rest and allow her body to heal properly. He prescribed stronger medication and his advice was: 'Let pain be your guide and rest as soon as it comes on'. He added that if there was no improvement at the end of another two weeks then he would arrange for an X-ray.

After two weeks there was still no improvement and she was now spending most of her time on the sofa watching television or reading. The normal pattern of life for the family was being disrupted. Ken was showing signs of fatigue and anxiety, not only about his wife but about neglecting work to give him more time at home. Colleagues who made allowances at first were now hinting that he was not pulling his weight. An sos was sent to Karen's retired parents to come and help out for a couple of weeks.

An appointment was made for Karen to have an X-ray – but two weeks ahead. By the time she went for her X-ray Karen had been away from work for six weeks and her condition showed no improvement. Yet another week went by while she waited for the results. Her doctor indicated that the X-ray showed no major problems except that '. . . there is a little bit of wear and tear which is to be expected when you get older, but this is nothing to worry about.' But, the doctor added, he would make an appointment for her to see a consultant orthopaedic surgeon at the hospital. In the meantime he advised continued rest and prescribed tranquilizers to calm her growing anxiety. By then it was July but holidays and a long waiting list meant that an appointment could not be arranged before the end of October!

During the waiting period Karen convinced herself that there was something seriously wrong which her doctor was keeping from her. This opinion was reinforced by the fact that she felt so weak. She soothed herself by nibbling constantly and she was putting on weight. She was feeling depressed and her hair was now lank and lifeless. The pain had now spread to her legs, shoulder and neck. Every movement provoked a pain spasm and she found it difficult to sleep. The family treated her as an invalid, fetching and carrying to save her getting out of her chair. Her parents' stay had become extended and Karen became more and more dependent on them. All her hobbies had been abandoned, along with shopping trips, meals out, weekend walks, taking the children to the swimming baths and youth clubs. Ken was more nurse than husband. They no longer had any physical closeness. Karen had lost interest and was totally concerned with her own pain and suffering. Ken was preoccupied with his own situation, having to share the house with in-laws, and cope with the pressures of having a sick wife. After the first month friends had drifted off and only telephoned occasionally to enquire about Karen's health. Anyone who did venture over the doorstep was given a blow-by-blow account of Karen's troubles.

Karen's employer, whilst sympathizing with her condition, regretted he had to find a full-time replacement. With the loss of her job, went Karen's company car. As a result of the added responsibility, Ken had turned down a promotion which would have meant him being away from home three nights a week. Without Karen's salary they were having to economize and their son's school trip to France had had to be abandoned.

The specialist's examination was inconclusive. He did not think there was a prolapsed disc or other structural problem. He said he would arrange for her to see a physiotherapist and review her situation after three months. 'In the meantime, just soldier on,' he said.

Five months had now elapsed since Karen's injury and she must now be considered to have joined the ranks of chronic pain sufferers. Over a period of six weeks she was given physiotherapy treatment to relax the muscles of her back and was given advice about posture and exercise. For a time the pain was easier but she still found movement painful, and because she was convinced that pain was synonymous with damage, she would not carry on doing the exercises once she got home.

Karen continued being treated as a complete invalid: she walked only if supported, spent most of her day with her feet up and she could no longer concentrate on reading. She went out only when taken in the car. Because of her disturbed nights Karen was also on sleeping tablets and had taken to sleeping downstairs so that Ken could get his rest. All decisions about the running of the house had been taken out of her hands. It now seemed to her that she was a burden to everybody and that they were caring for her less out of love than a sense of duty. She had long periods of silence and found herself crying from sheer frustration and had outbursts of temper over minor details, directed at those closest to her. Consequently the children escaped from home as often as possible to find relief from the gloomy atmosphere.

Karen and Ken were both convinced she was seriously ill and were frightened at the change that had come over her. On her second visit to the consultant she was in a sorry state. Together they challenged his diagnosis, insisting that there must be something seriously wrong with Karen. He had only to look at her! The consultant repeated that the tests so far showed no abnormalities, but he would arrange for her to go into hospital as a day patient to have a spinal injection to relieve the pain for a time so that she could 'get about more easily'.

Karen waited *another six weeks* before being called to the hospital but it was worth the wait. Quite soon after the injection she found that the pain was relieved and she could move freely. She celebrated her improvement by tackling some of the household jobs that had been neglected. Although the spirit was willing, the body was still weak. Muscles were wasted and she had lost her stamina. She pushed herself for a number of hours, and the result was that she strained her wasted muscles and became exhausted. A downcast Karen retired to bed for a few days to recover. This setback reinforced her belief that pain resulted from activity and that her efforts had caused further damage. She was soon back in the role of invalid and restricted her movement as much as possible.

When she next saw the consultant, three months after the injection, she was in a depressed state and even more convinced that there must be something seriously wrong with her. The consultant thought it might be useful to carry out a full body scan as this would give a clearer indication of any problems. However, they were warned to expect to wait up to *six months* as there was only one machine in the region. In fact Karen waited seven months.

During this time Karen continued resting and was supplied regularly with pain-killers, tranquilizers and sleeping tablets which she took conscientiously. Her daily intake was 14 assorted tablets.

Surely by now, she felt, her problem must be very obvious as she was almost completely disabled by her pain. Paradoxically the family was hoping that some disease or abnormality would be found to explain the pain so that an operation could be performed to put it right. Their feeling was that you could not have such pain without there being a cause and it was the doctors' responsibility to find that cause. How else could the problem be treated?

The results, however, were very different. The consultant was pleased to be able to tell them that there did not appear to be any sign of disease, abnormality or damage at all and that this should put their minds at rest. He would, however, make an appointment to review her case in six months time.

Instead of the news having the desired effect, the family was devastated and felt completely helpless. Imagine: Karen, crippled with pain, socially isolated, family relationships distorted, feeling completely demoralized and vulnerable, sitting in front of the consultant, looking 10 years older than her years, being asked to believe that there was nothing wrong with her – so far as they could tell! Karen had the impression that she was being told that her problem was a figment of her imagination. This impression was confirmed in her own mind when the consultant suggested that a chat with his colleague, a psychiatrist, might be helpful!!! She was now faced with three possibilities: (1) that there may still be some hidden physical cause for her pain, (2) that her pain was a product of her overactive imagination, or (3) that she was mentally ill. Alarm was now added to the already long list of difficulties facing her . . .

Here we have a youthful, energetic woman who has achieved as a wife and mother, holds down a responsible job and is socially outgoing. She has never faced serious illness before and is suddenly struck down.

Beware rest *does not turn into* rust

Initially Karen was advised by her doctor to go to bed for an indefinite period. Had the pain eased quickly then perhaps she could have regarded the incident as no more than an interruption to her normal life. However, Karen was given the vague instruction to rest 'until the pain eased'. The fact that she was left to determine the course of the illness for herself was not very helpful.

Very few instances of back pain, even those caused by injury, lead to disability, and recent research indicates that in the case of back injury, the recovery rate is enhanced if a doctor specifically advocates bed rest for one week only before gradually resuming normal activities. If at the same time the patient can be helped towards improving posture and doing appropriate exercise to strengthen the weakened muscles, then not only is the recovery quicker but there is also less chance of a recurrence in the future. Interestingly enough, when the doctor's instruction is to rest completely for two days only then the recovery rate is twice as good as when seven days is recommended. It is wiser, therefore, to specify a precise length of time for recovery. To leave it open-ended may be interpreted by the patient to mean that the future is uncertain and that it is important to guard against further injury by limiting activity. It is precisely this kind of approach which can result in the development of an over-protective attitude on the part of the patient and family and may play a major part in establishing the chronic pain state, contributing to disability and suffering over a long period. By following the instruction to 'let pain be your guide', Karen had learned to interpret feelings of discomfort and pain as indicators of yet unhealed or undiscovered injury or disease. As a result, her symptoms developed, not so much because of the original injury, but because of the oft'repeated prescription to rest she avoided movement as much as possible. When the body is not exercised then there is muscle wastage, the body becomes less efficient and limbs become painful, leading to more disuse, and more pain.

21

Communication problems

As we saw, Karen, her family – and her medical practitioners – believed that where there is pain, there must be a physical cause and that the severity of the pain must be related to the degree of injury, damage or abnormality. Conversely, if a physical cause cannot be found then the pain cannot be real and must be the product of the imagination. This is not so! Pain is not directly proportional to damage or injury.

Throughout, Karen had been in a considerable amount of confusion as a result of rather vague messages from the professionals.

The illness was never clearly identified to Karen (and this is very often difficult to do in the case of back pain) but at an early stage she could have been reassured that although her pain was really acute, there was no evidence of disease, or of nerve or tissue damage. It could have been explained that pain can continue for some time after healing has taken place and that pain on movement did not mean that she was doing herself any further injury. Her fear of further injury should have been recognized.

The communication from her doctor that the X-ray showed 'a little bit of wear and tear' related to the ageing process was probably meant to be helpful but in fact was misinterpreted and added to Karen's general anxiety. This unexpected traumatic episode happening in the prime of life is alarming, bringing with it reminders of mortality and unwanted messages about a possible bleak future. In fact X-rays of most adults approaching their forties will show some signs of wear and tear associated with ageing. Some people will show a great deal of wear and tear which produces no pain and no disability whatsoever whilst others have the pain with nothing to show for it.

In addition Karen was given the advice to 'soldier on' without a clear explanation of what was meant or any guidance on how she should do it. This is a phrase commonly used and causes a lot of confusion if it is left hanging in the air as it was in this case. It is being implied that the person is not being brave and must learn to grin and bear it.

Expectations

Throughout her contact with her medical advisers, Karen had repeatedly had her hopes raised, only to have them dashed, believing, like most of us, that when you consult a doctor with a problem it is his job to find the solution. In highly developed countries such as our own where there are sophisticated medical services, there is a tendency to surrender responsibility for our health to the professionals and to expect them to have an answer to every problem we hand over to them. Anyone with chronic pain must learn that if the pain is to be treated successfully then that person must play a leading role. Unfortunately, these lessons are hard to learn at a time of crisis especially when the professionals go on acting as though they know best! Karen was constantly being given mixed messages by the practitioners: they told her they could find nothing wrong and yet they were planning to carry out further examinations and tests. Each test built up hopes that at last the root of the problem would be found, and each time she was disappointed that no named illness was discovered which could be treated, and what is more, cured. Her expectations were at fever pitch over the scan. What must it be like to receive a message that the scan is clear and there is nothing to show the cause of the pain but that perhaps a psychiatrist is called for! Could it be that her pain results from the machinations of a sick mind?

Time heals all ills?!

The gaps between investigations, consultations and treatments were far too long. These allowed time for Karen and her family to make unhelpful adaptations. Fears were given time to ferment and nurture the chronic pain condition. There is nothing like fear and anxiety for wasting energy which could be used in the healing process. Fear and anxiety alone can be enough to produce helplessness and disability. In my own experience as a patient and as a therapist the treatment of fear and anxiety has to go hand in hand with treatment of the body.

Physiotherapy treatment came far too late in the day. Already Karen had developed a fear of movement ('motophobia'? I may be coining a new word) because of her belief that she might do herself an injury. Weekly appointments were insufficient to help Karen overcome this phobia. What she needed at this stage was daily attendance under supervision and encouragement to carry out the exercises necessary to strengthen her weakened muscles and improve her mobility.

The spinal injection which was intended to help, and did in fact bring some relief for a time, should have been linked to physiotherapy appointments and teaching about building up activity SLOWLY and progressively.

In fact, physiotherapy could have been offered at a much earlier stage involving a programme of gradually increasing exercise accompanied by massage, manipulation, heat treatment or ultrasound. But this would not necessarily guarantee that Karen would avoid chronic pain. No one knows why it begins in each individual case. We still have to take into account the shock of realizing that one is vulnerable to physical problems and the impact of this on the personality.

Medication can add to the problem

Already we have seen that chronic pain reduces a person's ability to function in many areas of life. You may be facing the realization that little likelihood exists that your underlying condition can be 'cured'. At this stage, the last thing you could wish for is to be on drugs which impair your ability to think clearly, make decisions and to take the necessary steps to regain control over your life. Anyone who suffers from chronic pain is likely to have some fantasy that somewhere there is a perfect pill which provides pain relief and yet has no unpleasant or long-lasting side effects.

There are many drugs and pain-killers which are useful for pain relief in the short term. Most of the proprietary drugs advertised nightly on television probably fall into this category and are useful for the occasional headache, toothache, muscle strain, and to ease pains associated with short-term illness. A number of drugs have been developed which are particularly effective for treating post-operative pain and for treating acute pain but the appropriate use of drugs in these situations is very different in the case of chronic pain.

In developing your own self-help strategy you need to have some understanding about the kinds of medication used in the treatment of pain.

The most powerful pain-killers are based on morphine or codeine and are often used effectively for post-operative pain over a very short period, or in the treatment of terminal cancer. There is a danger of addiction from these drugs and it is also likely that ever-increasing doses are needed to control the pain. It is easy to become tolerant to these drugs thus making them less effective. Obviously, these are not recommended for chronic pain.

Anyone with chronic pain is likely to have other analgesics or muscle-relaxants prescribed. They are effective, however, for only a mild amount of pain and increasing the dosage can often produce stomach upset, constipation, or more seriously, liver or kidney damage. Those drugs based on paracetamol are not likely to have an effect on inflammatory conditions. Aspirin-like drugs and other non-steroidal anti-inflammatory drugs (NSAIDs) are useful for low levels of pain and for reducing inflammation in conditions like arthritis. Unfortunately, not everyone can tolerate aspirin which can upset the stomach or cause ulcers. In their favour, such drugs are not addictive but because they are mild analgesics there is the danger that long-lasting high levels of pain will be treated with increased doses thereby increasing the likelihood of harmful side-effects.

Steroids are also used to reduce inflammation but these are not to be advised for chronic pain except in the most severe cases of rheumatoid arthritis.

There is evidence that many chronic pain patients have become addicted and toxic from the protracted use of painkillers and muscle relaxants including tranquilizers. Further, research indicates that these drugs and sedative hypnotic drugs, in particular Valium and Librium, can be responsible for causing chronic pain. In many cases doing nothing more than ceasing medication and increasing activity levels can eliminate the distress of chronic pain. Unfortunately we live in a society which places an over-reliance on drugs. Patients go to see a medical practitioner expecting to be given drugs of one kind or another whatever the problem. Self-medication has been encouraged and pharmaceutical companies compete with attractive advertising and slogans for the most effective pain-killers. People will often supplement tablets from the doctor with over-the-counter pills thus increasing the chances of developing toxicity. There still persists in the minds of lay people (and many professionals) the idea that if there is a pain it can be alleviated by drugs no matter how long the pain has persisted, and that the answer to intractable pain is to increase the dosage. Any drugs likely to be used over a long period should be avoided if they cause sedation, addiction, toxicity, depression, digestive/liver/and kidney upsets, or bleeding.

Perhaps it is appropriate then, to think about the part that drugs played in establishing and maintaining Karen's chronic pain and disability. In the early stages Karen, quite rightly, was given pain-killers and muscle relaxants to help reduce her pain and take away the tension in the muscles. However, these tablets were continued over a long period and the dosage increased, even though they were providing no perceptible pain relief.

Anxiety in patients with chronic pain is common and as stress and anxiety are contributors to pain, it may seem appropriate that tranquilizers are used. However, in long term use (i.e. over a matter of months) such drugs may exacerbate the pain problem. The drugs are addictive, cause sleep disturbance and tend to contribute to depression. Since depression is a likely result of chronic pain anyway, then it is better to avoid such medication. Tranquilizers not only relax the painful muscles in the short term but influence the brain in such a way that it inhibits its ability to produce endorphins, the body's own natural painkillers. If you also take into account that such drugs produce drowsiness, affect memory and concentration and increase fatigue, then you have other reasons for avoiding them. Sometimes tranquilizers may be given to reduce cramps and spasms. They may be helpful if used for short periods in acute conditions but they are not appropriate for long-term use especially when the aim is to help the patient relax tight muscles. This can be done much more effectively by learning a few simple relaxation skills. Karen's problem was further compounded by the fact that she had been prescribed sleeping tablets.

Illness strikes at the whole person . . .

To complete this analysis it is important to highlight the emotional response of Karen herself and to examine the role of her family during this difficult period in their lives. The sudden attack to

Karen's body produced both a physical and emotional shock. The central core of her being was deeply wounded. Her confidence was shattered, her stature in the world of business, as a parent, as a wife, as a member of a community, was reduced, and therefore as a person she was diminished. Little wonder she developed a negative view of herself and her ability to change her circumstances. This is often the result of chronic pain and unfortunately the negativity can make the pain worse. Add to this, anxiety about the seriousness of her condition, loss of income, loss of prestige, loss of friends and workmates and a feeling that she was no longer attractive, then we have a situation which increases tension and in turn increases the pain. She had ceased to have any fun in her life.

Fun and positive experiences have a direct influence on a person's experience of pain. Anyone who is enjoying themselves has less pain. Unfortunately, the psychology of Karen had been overlooked in the attempt to find the cause and cure for her pain. At the end of the investigations we found Karen grieving for her past and lost future. Her feeling of helplessness – probably the most serious illness a person can have – produced an inability to believe that she had any control over her own life and she had this real fear that she would never be able to function normally again. Between herself and her loved ones there developed a wall of separation which prevented any constructive discussion focusing on her real feelings and fears. She shared with many chronic pain sufferers the feeling that decisions were being made behind her back, secrets being kept from her, and yet she dreaded knowing what they were.

. . . and the family

Karen had a supportive family during her sickness but we have to question at what point family support ceases to be helpful and begins to limit the patient's recovery and increase dependence. In Karen's case she was surrounded by a concerned family, eager to help and probably unused to the mainstay of the family being ill. The illness may have been a godsend to her retired parents who wanted something to do to prove their continuing worth to the family and to use up their own excess energy. The end result is a family of six helpless people all sharing the problem and unable to do anything about it.

27

Some parts of Karen's story may strike a chord and echo some of your own feelings about the treatment you have received as you have progressed towards the chronic pain state. In the beginning, like me, you put your faith in the doctors and were reassured that in time things would get better. But, as time went on, and anxiety grew, fears increased, and confusion took over, and you lost confidence. You may even have developed feelings of antipathy, frustration and anger towards those qualified people whom you felt MUST know all about your problem . . . and the way to cure it! Like Karen, you were right to expect prompt and effective treatment and to expect that the professionals would be aware of the impact the illness was having on you as a person. With hindsight, do you think that perhaps you were expecting too much of the medical profession? Did you get the impression that when your pain state reached chronic proportions it was no longer worth trying to reverse it? Do you still think it cannot be reversed?

There is a form of treatment called 'Pain Management' that tackles every aspect of this problem which affects the body, mind and spirit and aims to galvanize patients to the point of taking the first step towards recovery and subsequently complete charge of their continuing progress.

3

The Way Out

One of the aims of this book is to inform you of the importance of developing pain management centres which are accessible to anyone who wants to control their pain and improve their quality of life. Pain management centres are indicative of the new approach which has been developed, mainly in the United States and Canada but simultaneously at Walton Hospital in Liverpool. The focus is on Pain Management and is based on the understanding that pain is not merely a physical problem. There are also programmes at St Thomas's Hospital, London, and other centres. They bring together, in one centre, resources which enable patients to receive a variety of treatments for pain relief and more than that, they are taught the skills to help themselves and to accept that managing pain can be a full-time occupation, prerequisite to the enjoyment of an enhanced quality of life. These centres provide a multi-faceted approach to pain management by bringing together practitioners from a variety of backgrounds, medical, psychological, complementary medicine, and even in some cases using the resources of former patients who are coping successfully with their own pain.

Pain relief clinics are available now to most people throughout the UK and during the last ten years Regional Hospital Boards have taken responsibility for establishing specialist units. Pain relief clinics, whilst recognizing that pain needs to be treated as an entity, focus primarily on the physical aspects of the problem and treatment options are taken in turn until the patient shows improvement.

In these centres it is recognized that pain is an illness in itself, needing specialized treatment, irrespective of its cause, and they are usually staffed by medical practitioners such as anaesthetists and neurologists, supported by psychologists, physiotherapists and occupational therapists who all understand the complex nature of chronic pain. Anyone who has persistent pain which is affecting the quality of their life and causing emotional and behavioural changes can be referred to a Pain Relief Clinic for an assessment. Usually treatment is given on an out-patient basis unless specific procedures are needed which can only be carried out in hospital.

There is bound to be some local variation in the style and treatment offered by these clinics according to the available resources but the one thing they have in common is the belief that pain exists irrespective of its source. It is likely that you will start by being given a full physical examination and be asked about your medical history, the history of your pain problem and your treatment to date. You may also be asked to fill in a questionnaire concerning the effects of your pain on your way of life, and on your relationships. You might be asked to undergo further tests and investigations and as a result of all these you should be able to have a full discussion with the staff about your problem and the treatment options.

Because of the medical orientation of most pain relief clinics you will probably be offered appropriate medication for your condition – for example, anti-inflammatory drugs, analgesics, anti-depressants and/or anti-convulsants. The fact that you may receive an anti-depressant does not mean that you are being treated for depression. There are certain pain conditions which respond well when anti-depressant medication is combined with anti-convulsants which can inhibit the haphazard firing of nerve impulses and may be contributing to your pain.

Another option which may be used separately or in conjunction with drugs is that of injections or nerve blocks. They are not intended as a cure but as part of your treatment programme. They are designed to interrupt the pain–spasm–pain cycle in order to give sufficient short-term relief from the pain. Sometimes a local anaesthetic is injected at the actual site of the pain or it may be injected in such a way as to block the nerve impulses carrying the pain message. An example of such a block is a steroid injection into the epidural space surrounding the spinal cord and nerves and this can be particularly helpful in the treatment of sciatica.

This treatment enables some people to become sufficiently mobile to take up their normal work and the restored activity may be enough for them to continue without further treatment. For those less fortunate it gives a breathing space to learn exercise techniques, relaxation skills and to participate in other active therapies with a reasonable degree of comfort.

The medical practitioner responsible for your treatment may also arrange for you to have physiotherapy and to receive advice on such matters as posture, lifting and exercise.

Sometimes you may be referred to a psychologist to learn relaxation and stress management techniques or to talk over some of your anxieties which may be resulting from, or contributing to your pain.

You may be referred to a psychiatrist and this is not to suggest that you are mentally ill, or that your problem is all in the mind. The purpose of such a referral is to check out the degree of distress or depression which you might have and to see whether you need some help over the short term to enable you to go forward with your treatment.

Although pain relief centres do provide a valuable service and are instrumental in ensuring that the majority of pain sufferers have their problem eased and they prevent a significant number from reaching a disabled state, there are many whose pain remains intractable. These are the people who need something more and this is where pain management comes into its own.

The pain management approach acknowledges that pain can quickly lead to total disability, disintegration of the personality and distorted personal relationships. The aim, therefore, is to provide within a three or four-week programme an opportunity for the patient to become reactivated and stronger, released from drug domination, skilled in self-help relaxation techniques, made aware of changes in attitudes and behaviour which have resulted from pain and learn new methods of relating to others. The patient is recognized as being a whole person who needs to be restored physically, emotionally and spiritually in order to cope with every aspect of life whilst carrying the burden of chronic pain.

As a patient on such a programme you will be encouraged to change your attitude and become an active participant in your own rehabilitation rather than the passive recipient of medical care which you may have become.

A pain management programme usually caters for a group of seven or eight patients at a time who will work together encouraging and supporting each other through the process of rehabilitation and learning. They meet every weekday from 9.00 a.m. till 5.00 p.m. approximately. The programme at Walton Hospital, Liverpool is an out-patient programme although others may be held on an in-patient basis. Having had experience of successful in-patient and out-patient programmes, my personal preference is the out-patient one which enables people to live at home or in lodgings in the vicinity of the hospital but away from institutional surroundings. The daily attendance provides an opportunity to get back into a work routine of getting up early, travelling to and from work and sustaining energy and interest throughout the day. This gives the patient a sense of normality and provides an opportunity to try out new learning immediately in their day-to-day contacts. As an in-patient you have to fit into a hospital routine and there is a possibility of separating out the hospital experience from the reality of life outside. At some point this has to be faced.

Of course the content of any programme will vary from hospital to hospital according to resources and the philosophy of those running the programme. Most, however, provide a common core of experience for the patients. Emphasis is placed on progressive exercise and improving mobility. A variety of relaxation techniques will be taught as well as guidance about using them to cope with everyday situations. Various aspects of behaviour which might be said to be unhelpful will be targeted for change by the patient and the group and staff together will monitor each patient's progress.

Understanding the problem of pain is an essential part of learning for each patient and instruction about drugs and their effects will be provided along with help for those wishing to wean themselves away from drug treatments. In some programmes there are opportunities for family members to take part in certain activities so that they, too, can understand the process.

It is also possible for a programme to help each patient face up to the prospect of returning to work, providing an assessment of ability and counselling about prospects, taking into account the length of absence from work and the physical stamina involved.

On the pain programme based in Seattle in the University of Washington Hospital, arrangements were made for some patients to continue their rehabilitation on a 'job station'. These were part-time unpaid jobs set up in various parts around the university campus. They were used for two purposes, (1) to help those planning to return to employment to try out different kinds of work to get a sense of how they 'fit' and (2) for those people not planning to return to work but needing a way of trying out different kinds of physical and social activities.

Although no official 'job station' exists at Walton, a number of patients are asked to volunteer to help in the day-to-day running of the pain management programme. Others are encouraged to seek new work opportunities or even set up self-help groups for people with pain in areas not served by a pain management programme.

My own experience in working with patients shows that it is possible for most people to achieve a high degree of skill in managing their pain without dependence on drugs. They can regain mobility, confidence and self-esteem, and go on to maintain their progress even to the extent of making useful voluntary contributions to the workforce or establishing themselves in a new career. This is remarkable as most people who attend a pain management programme have been written off as hopeless cases.

The remaining chapters therefore will help you, step by step, to develop your own resources in order to regain control over your pain and your own life. You can do this provided you accept that your problem has taken time to develop, it has been with you a long time, and it will take time to sort out. This means dedicating yourself to following the exercise and relaxation programmes every day – for the rest of your life!

Some other aids to relieving pain

Electrical stimulators (TENS)

Many people are helped by a small battery-operated device which transmits electrical impulses through wires to electrodes attached to the skin near the painful area. This is known as a Transcutaneous Electrical Nerve Stimulator (TENS). The unit is simple and easy to use and even when used over long periods has been found to be safe, and if used as directed, has no harmful side effects. When the unit is turned on, the machine produces an electrical tingling sensation, the strength and frequency of which can be increased or decreased by the user according to the severity of the pain.

The practice of using electrical stimulation for the treatment of pain is not new. It is said to date back to Roman times when electric eels would be wrapped around the ankle of a patient while standing in wet sand. This treatment was said to be an effective cure for headaches! I can remember from my own childhood my grandfather's highly polished wooden box which contained apparatus for producing electrical impulses. The patient held on to brass grips and when a handle on the side of the box was turned received a mild shock said to be an effective treatment for nervous disorders. TENS is rather more sophisticated and is designed to work on the principle of the gate control theory referred to earlier (see p. 12). Put simply, the electrical impulse, through the skin, is transmitted over the large nerve fibres (the fast route) thus blocking out the transmissions from the small nerve fibres (the slow route) which are transmitting pain. The pain sensation is replaced by a tingling sensation.

Research suggests that TENS may also work because the tingling sensation distracts the person's attention from the pain sensation or alternatively the stimulation helps the release of endorphins in the brain and spinal cord. You will remember that endorphins are natural pain-killers produced in the body.

Not everyone obtains relief by means of TENS but it is worth discussing its suitability for you with your medical practitioner. Recent research indicates that up to one-third of people using TENS find it helpful. Several short trials lasting half an hour or so will be enough to let you know if the machine is suitable for you. Some people find that brief periods of stimulation can bring about pain relief for a matter of hours, days or even longer. Others need to wear the device throughout their waking hours in order to obtain relief. The great advantage of TENS is that, once you have been shown how to use it, you can carry on using it and experiment in finding the point on your body which gives you the greatest amount of relief and you can vary the controls at any time according to your need. It is possible to switch off the machine altogether whilst still leaving the electrodes attached. It is then ready for use when you require it.

Many people find that the device enables them to cut out completely the use of drugs and in my own case, because of the adverse reactions I experience with anti-inflammatory drugs and pain-killers, I find TENS safe, reliable and effective and I would always prefer to use TENS as a first-choice pain-reliever as it enables me to maintain a level of activity which I could not possibly achieve any other way. Some people are advised to use the machine when pain dictates but I prefer to put the machine on first thing in the morning when dressing as this is the most convenient time. I find that small amounts of stimulation before the pain sets in can be much more effective than waiting until the pain has started in earnest. However, if you use one, you may find that your pattern of use is quite different; you have to find the way that suits you best.

The minor disadvantages of using TENS are outweighed by the benefits it brings. Prolonged use can bring about a skin irritation around the site of the electrodes. There are various kinds of tapes and pads for attaching the electrodes to the skin and it is worthwhile experimenting with these. The skin irritations can be avoided provided the electrodes are not always placed on the same site and that after use, the skin is washed thoroughly and a little moisturizing lotion is applied. If you find that TENS gives you the power to control your pain then do not be put off by this minor nuisance. If you attend a pain clinic as an out-patient you may be offered one to try out and then be given details of how and where to purchase the machine. So far as I know these machines are not yet available free of charge through the NHS even though the cost of supplying and maintaining a patient on one of these machines would be considerably less than maintaining the same patient on drugs over a long period.

If you are not attending a pain clinic then you should ask your doctor where you can buy a TENS machine. The machine MUST be used under medical supervision and in the interests of safety it must not be used if you are wearing a heart pacemaker, when bathing, near microwave ovens, whilst sleeping, or driving. The machine is light and designed to fit into a pocket or on a belt. It is no more obvious than wearing a telephone paging unit and will not interfere with normal movements.

It is important, however, that you do not simply sit back and allow TENS to do the work of controlling your pain on its own. The machine works best in conjunction with your dedication to improving your mobility, strengthening exercises, relaxation techniques and extending your range of physical and social activities generally.

Surgery

There are cases where surgery is an essential part of the treatment of pain, particularly where material from a ruptured disc presses on nerves and surrounding tissues causing pain and serious dysfunction in other parts of the body.

In recent years a technique has been developed whereby ruptured discs are dissolved with injections of a chemical called chymopapain although this treatment is less traumatic than surgery, there is a small risk of allergic reaction and a great deal of care is taken before deciding whether or not this method is appropriate.

Surgery may also be carried out where the actual nerves carrying the pain messages to the brain have been severed in order to bring some relief. This may not always bring permanent relief as nerves can be regenerated, but even if relief is provided only for a short time it gives the patient an opportunity to learn other methods of pain management.

Surgery should only be recommended as a last resort and should never be used as a first-choice option. The more often a person has surgery for pain, the less chance there is of achieving positive results.

Acupuncture

Pain clinics may also make use of acupuncture which involves the manipulation of very fine needles at specific points on the skin. Like TENS it is suggested that acupuncture helps the stimulation of the large nerve fibres thus preventing signals from the small pain-carrying fibres reaching the brain, or alternatively, that acupuncture stimulates the release of the body's own painkillers, endorphins.

4

Exercise

Do not be tempted to skip this chapter! It is probably the most important chapter in the book for anyone concerned with managing their pain and getting back to enjoying an increased quality of life. Many patients suffering from pain are advised to rest if pain results from movement. There is a temptation for people in pain to tense their muscles and hold them rigidly. For this reason, in acute pain conditions, it is sensible to rest as movement at an early stage after injury can further aggravate torn muscles, ligaments, or discs which are swollen and inflamed. This advice is also valid in the case of arthritis sufferers going through a period of severe inflammation in the joints. In order to allow maximum healing to take place naturally, one or two weeks' rest is recommended, along with a course of pain-killers. It is then possible to get back gradually to normal healthy functioning.

Pain which continues for three months, or longer, enters the chronic phase, and if allowed to go untreated can have serious physical, psychological and social consequences. It is vital that this should not happen and the most effective way of prevention is to take up a programme of exercise which will gradually increase mobility, flexibility and circulation. Arthritis sufferers in particular need exercise to strengthen, condition and maintain a range of motion in the joints and to manage the pain.

Your medical advisers will confirm the appropriate time to start exercising.

But first of all, let's look at what happens when we do not exercise . . .

The experience of pain over a period of time reduces the amount of exercise we take and muscles which have been inactive become atrophied and weak, becoming shorter and therefore more likely to go into spasm. This process of weakening can take place relatively quickly. If you have ever broken an arm or leg you will remember just how thin and wasted the limb appeared when the plaster was removed and that you were probably given physiotherapy for some time to help restore the limb to normal functioning. The person with chronic pain is in danger of facing this deterioration throughout the whole body, irrespective of the seat of the pain, because the general level of activity becomes greatly reduced.

In my own case, I virtually lost all mobility – I found it difficult to turn my head, it was painful to support a book or even to grasp a knife or fork. The condition may be exacerbated by shortage of breath and a feeling of weakness and fatigue when attempting movement. Not only will the muscles of the arms, legs and trunk be affected but the efficiency of the heart and lungs is also likely to suffer.

Many people recognize the importance of exercise but are tempted to do too much or do the wrong kind. This can be very harmful, producing exhaustion, pulled muscles and an intolerably increased level of pain. And this experience will only increase the conviction that pain is synonymous with movement. If this has happened to you, no doubt you have become frustrated, angry, irritable and most likely, depressed, and decide that it is better to rest than damage yourself further by continuing any activity at all. You may even develop a fear about movement which may become so strong that it grows into a phobia. Anyone who has this condition, which I shall call 'motophobia', will need a great deal of convincing that no harm will come from moving around.

You may therefore feel very resistant to the idea of exercise. You are not alone in having these feelings. I myself was convinced that movement, because it was painful, would damage me further. Like many others I had been told repeatedly to rest if I felt pain and to get used to leading a completely restricted life. The whole idea of exercise was frightening and my first physiotherapy session on the pain management programme produced feelings of intense anger. Like others in the group, I regarded the physiotherapist with all the loathing that one might feel towards a mediaeval torturer! She became the focus for all my rage, frustration and bad feelings which stemmed from losing many of the things that were important to me.

My first attempts at exercise were, to say the least, reluctant and I grudgingly set a target of one for each of the required exercises. I would have preferred not to do any! During the first week I continued to resist and did not raise my target above one on any day. By the following week I had had a chance to think things over and to absorb the message that PAIN DOES NOT NECESSARILY EQUATE WITH DAMAGE OR INJURY.

More importantly, I had learned that unless I moved I would permanently lose the ability to move. Also, I had a strong feeling that even the feeble attempts I had made had produced some improvement in my condition. I was later to find that my experience was shared by many of the patients undergoing this programme of physical reactivation.

During the second week I increased my targets and by the end of a month I was completing 30 repetitions of every exercise daily and was ready for more! By that time I was thoroughly convinced that exercise was having a direct influence on the frequency and severity of my pain and that I could make it work for me as a form of pain-killer.

Movement is the key to rehabilitation, to getting fit, to managing pain and to resuming your normal lifestyle. Research shows that exercise stimulates the production of endorphins, a natural chemical produced by the body. This has the effect of inducing a feeling of well-being and has a direct influence on reducing pain. Conversely therefore, inactivity results in a low level of endorphins in the bloodstream and reduces the body's capacity to cope with pain and the resulting depression.

Some guidelines

There are certain principles which you need to follow in an exercise programme. The main aim of any exercise is that it should:

- **Condition the whole body**
- **Be regular and controlled** and should aim at building up strength, stamina and increasing mobility.

What's more:

- **Exercise should not involve strain**: it is important to remember that your body is being retrained, so exercising to the point of over-tiredness must be avoided. Even gentle exercise may produce some aches and pains afterwards but these are nothing to worry about. Gradually, you will find that you are able to extend yourself a little more but in the early stages just go gently and avoid becoming too ambitious.

39

- **Steady and positive progress needs to be rewarded**: increasing strength and mobility are rewards in themselves but take pride in your achievement and reward yourself with treats at various steps along the way.

Before starting your course of exercise, make out a simple record, starting with your present daily activity level over the past week. Note particularly the amount of time you spend sitting, reclining or lying down. Compare this with the amount of time spent on your feet walking, standing, preparing meals and doing other tasks. Maintain this chart for reference and continue to keep it regularly so that you can check your progress. Your aim is to spend proportionally more time in activity than in rest. Therefore, any activity which leads towards this goal is beneficial.

- **It is important that you get advice about what is appropriate exercise for you**: your GP can advise you directly or put you in touch with a physiotherapist, or you may enlist the help of the specialist staff at your local sports centre in devising a course of exercises specific to your needs. Some other forms of exercise which you may find helpful are swimming (a physiotherapist will no doubt be able to suggest a range of pool exercises for developing muscle strength and mobility). An advantage of exercising in the water is that the weight of the body is supported. Water exercise is therefore to be recommended even for non-swimmers. Hatha Yoga, Tai' Chi and dancing are all helpful in providing enjoyable progressive forms of exercise in a social context.

Outlined below are some examples of exercises which are used on the Pain Management Programme at Walton Hospital, Liverpool. Although the exercises in themselves do not take very long, it is a good idea to spread them out over a period of half an hour. At the beginning this will allow you to take things slowly and steadily and to rest between exercises. As you make progress and become stronger, more mobile and less fatigued, you will find that the whole period will be taken up by the exercises themselves. Half-an-hour each day is sufficient. Personally, I find it helpful to do the exercise in the morning as a way of warming up and getting muscles stretched in preparation for the day's activities. It is always useful to follow the exercise session with a period of deep relaxation. Relaxation is easier to achieve following exercise.

- **It is important to set yourself targets for each exercise** and to increase the target daily: aim to make steady, positive progress without becoming strained or over-tired. If at any time, as a result of over-enthusiasm, you set a target for the day which is beyond you, don't be put off – just adjust your target to a comfortable level and build up again.
- **Be content with steady progress and reward your achievements**: the important thing is to enjoy the movement and to succeed. It is a well-known fact that a small success in one area of our life can breed sufficient confidence to enable us to go on to succeed at other things. Although I give suggested initial targets for these exercises, you may set a target higher or lower than that suggested according to your level of mobility.

Exercises that can be done lying down

1. Ankle and calf stretch (this exercise can also be done in a sitting position.)

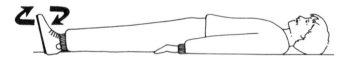

Rotate each ankle in turn slowly, first clockwise, then anticlockwise.

Initial target 5 times in each direction.

2. Foot stretch

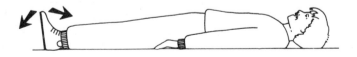

With both legs extended in front of you, point toes towards the

41

ceiling then, bending from ankle, move your toes away from you.
Now bending at the ankle, bring your toes towards you as far as you
can. Initial target 5 repetitions of these movements.

3. Pelvic tilt

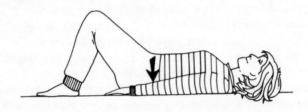

Lie on your back with knees bent. By tightening your lower
abdominal muscles, press your lower back flat against the floor.
Hold for 5 seconds. Repeat until you reach the target set.

Initial target 5 repetitions.

If you have back problems, then this exercise is a MUST and you
will benefit by practising this exercise several times a day.

4. Hip stretch

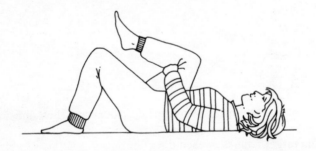

Lying on your back with knees bent, place both hands under your
right knee and gently raise it towards your chest, keeping your back
flat on the floor. Hold that position for about 5 seconds then gently
lower the leg to the floor. Repeat with the left leg. Initial target 5
repetitions for each leg.

5. Double knee to chest

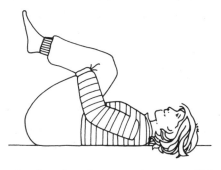

With both hands placed under your knees, pull knees to chest keeping your lower back flat on the floor. Hold for 5 seconds. This exercise gives a more complete stretch to the lower back and hip muscles.

Initial target 5 repetitions.

6. Half press-up

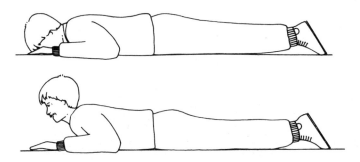

Lying on your stomach, facing forward, legs slightly apart in a relaxed position, bend the arms and place your hands on the floor level with your ears. Pressing down on your hands and forearms, gently raise your shoulders a few inches off the floor. At this stage do not straighten the arms completely. Keep your stomach and lower part of your body on the floor.

Initial target 5 repetitions.

The cat

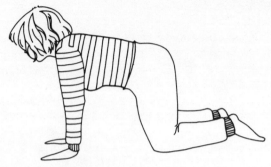

(fig. a)

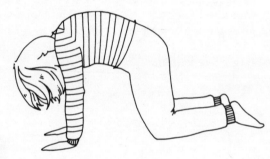

(fig. b)

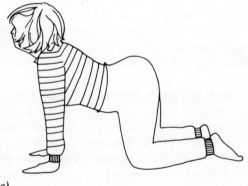

(fig. c)

7. The cat

Kneel on all-fours, knees and hands slightly apart with your spine in a straight line with the floor (fig. a). Breathe in, and as you do so, arch your back and bring your head down towards your chest allowing your head to follow the curve of the arch (fig. b). Then, slowly breathe out and hollow your back, at the same time raising your head as far as possible (fig. c). Look up and hold this position for 5 seconds.

Initial target 5 repetitions.

8. Hamstring stretch

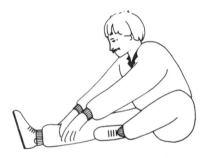

Sit with both legs extended and with back straight (if sitting in this way is difficult then sit with your back against a wall or door). Bend your left leg and place your left foot along the inside of your right thigh. Bending from the hips, reach forward with both hands to grasp your right leg as near to the ankle as possible and hold for 5 seconds. Straighten up slowly.

Repeat 5 times for each leg.

Exercises in a standing position

1. Knee raising

Standing straight, with feet slightly apart. If you are unsure of your balance, hold on to a support. Bend the right knee and bring it up towards your chest. Lower to the floor and repeat with the left leg.

Initial target 5 repetitions for each leg.

45

2. Arm circling

Stand with your feet slightly apart and your arms down by your side. Keeping the right arm straight, raise it and take it back in a full circle, brushing your ear with your upper arm. Repeat with the left arm.

Initial target 5 repetitions each arm.

3. Push-aways

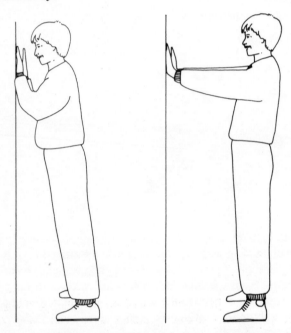

Stand with your feet slightly apart at arms reach from a wall. Put your hands against the wall at shoulder height. Keeping your back and legs straight, lean forward until your chest comes near the wall. Now, push away until you are back in the starting position. Initial target 5 repetitions.

4. Step-ups

Using a doorstep or bottom step of the stairs, step up with the right foot, bring the left foot on to the step alongside the right foot and step down with the right foot followed by the left foot. Repeat until the target is achieved. Now go through the process again beginning with the left foot.

Initial target 5 repetitions each side.

5. *Wall slide*

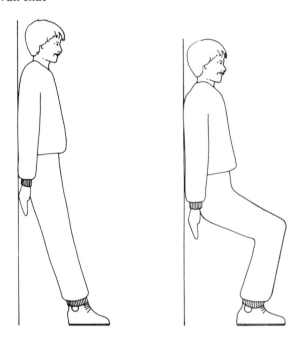

Stand with your back flat against a wall or door with feet slightly apart with your heels about 9 inches away from the wall. Slowly bend the knees and keeping your back firmly against the wall, slide up and down, pushing with your leg muscles.

Initial target 5 repetitions.

6. *Side stretch*

Stand with your feet slightly apart and hands hanging loosely by your sides. Bending slowly sideways to the right, let your right hand move down your thigh as far as comfortable. Hold this position for 5 seconds then slowly straighten up.

Repeat 5 times to the right and then to the left.

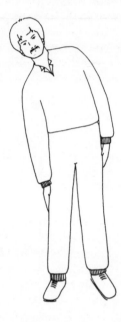

There are many other exercises which are invaluable for people with arthritis, knee problems and neck problems and it is strongly advisable to seek specialist advice on appropriate exercises for these areas. I have limited my suggestions to those exercises which are suitable for general strengthening, flexibility and conditioning for the majority of people, regardless of age or physical condition. If you have trouble walking normally because of your pain and you have got into the habit of limping, stooping, shuffling, or 'list' to one side, or if you have taken to using a walking stick, you may need some help to change your pattern of walking. Making the change is not as difficult as it might seem. 'Speed walking' is an excellent way to regain a more normal gait. Measure out a distance, for example, 25 or 50 yards and time yourself, or get someone else to do it, as you walk over the area as quickly as possible. There is no special place to do this. You might like to try it using the distance between two lamp-posts. Make a note of the time achieved and continue repeating the same walk daily and you will see a distinct improvement in the time taken. You will also find that your walking becomes smoother and more rhythmic. It helps to have spectators on the sideline to cheer you on! Not only does this exercise help you to break old walking habits, it is also an excellent aerobic exercise – that is, it helps you to take more oxygen into your body, thus increasing the efficiency of your heart and lungs. Whenever you are walking outdoors remember to vary your pace frequently especially if you find you are beginning to dawdle or shuffle.

Posture

I have found that many people with pain problems have difficulty in accepting that bad posture can actually cause their pain or at least can be a contributory factor. During the working day a driver can spend many hours in a driving seat which is badly designed or not correctly adjusted. What happened to ergonomics? People working at benches or worktops may stand up for long periods at a work surface of the wrong height (kitchen unit manufacturers please note!). Hairdressers and dentists, for example, stand for long periods exerting a strain on neck, shoulder and arm muscles. Supermarket checkout staff have to make movements to one side of the body only, and in a very limited space. Even at home it is possible to sit or recline in a comfortable armchair or settee for up to 5 hours at a time without proper back or head support and then go to bed to sleep with too many pillows, on a sagging or an over-firm mattress.

Anyone who maintains one position for long periods, or has bad posture, is likely to be prone to cricks in the neck and muscular spasm arising from excessive tension.

Bad posture is known to be the main reason for neck pain. Sitting or standing in a slouched position with the chin jutted forward, flattens the normal cervical curve in the neck, putting a strain on all the muscles supporting the head. Sleeping with too many pillows has the same effect so that the head is pushed forward throughout the night. Conversely, many people stand, walk, sit or sleep in positions which thrust the head backwards, lifting the chin up.

Bad posture may be the result of injury or, possibly, foot problems which throw the body out of alignment and place undue tension on individual muscles or groups of muscles in one part of the body. The body operates on a simple mechanical process involving action and reaction. Quite simply, if you stretch an elastic band, placing it under tension, it springs back into place when the tension is relaxed. The same happens with healthy muscles which are designed to stretch or contract and return to a normal resting state. However, if you maintain the tension in the elastic band for a long period then the band loses its elasticity and does not return to its normal shape. A similar thing happens when muscles are over-stretched and kept under tension for long periods. Holding the tension can produce pain and discomfort and the release of tension causes the muscle to go into spasm in its efforts to get back to normal. This is very painful.

You will know all about this if you have chronic pain. You will also know that your posture has probably suffered as a result of trying to find the least painful positions. You may have become used to sitting with one leg extended stiffly in front of you or to one side whilst your body leans over or twists. As you rise from your chair you may have developed the habit of holding your back or side and maintaining a stooped-over position as you walk away from the chair. This is known as 'guarding' behaviour, a tendency to want to protect the painful part. When challenged, like most of us, you will probably defend this behaviour, saying that you feel comfortable doing this, and that to sit, stand or walk any other way produces extreme discomfort and even pain. This is not surprising if your 'guarding' behaviour is of long standing and you have held various muscle groups in your body under tension to form a protective 'splint' around the original pain source. If you do not believe that your body has become distorted then look in a mirror when sitting or standing. See whether your head tilts one way or the other; is your chin raised? are your shoulders hunched? are you leaning forward or perhaps sideways from the waist? are you walking on the outside of your foot? Better still, ask your partner, or best friend, to give you some feedback on your posture.

Correcting your posture

Changes to posture will often bring about quite dramatic improvements in the frequency and severity of pain. Exercises designed to tone, stretch and strengthen your muscles will help but improvement will only be maintained if you become aware of the habits you have developed and seek to change them. You are not going to do

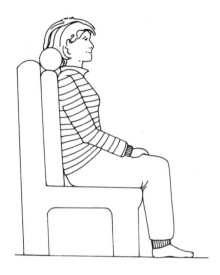

this all at once. I have only recently become aware that I have always had a tendency to allow my head to drop back and my chin to tilt up, thus aggravating the disc problem in my neck so in recent weeks I have consciously checked the way I hold my head when sitting, standing, walking and lying down and made the necessary adjustments. I have always considered myself a slow learner as far as posture is concerned. It has taken me a long time to understand what is meant by good posture. The words that people use to describe good posture can be misunderstood. Personally I find a visual demonstration more effective. So I will attempt to use as few words as possible in explaining how to develop good posture. The illustration above shows how to sit correctly so that the whole body is in a state of balance.

Your head and neck

Correcting head and neck posture is quite simple and needs very few words. Just check when you are sitting, standing or walking that your chin remains parallel to the floor, not tilted up, not dropped forward, and with eyes looking straight ahead. At the same time notice whether there is any tension in your shoulders and allow them to relax and drop. There is a tendency when reading, to lower the head, putting a strain on the muscles at the back of the neck. Many modern chairs are low-backed and these are to be avoided when sitting for long spells. If you find yourself sitting in a high-backed chair which does not allow you to keep your head in the right position, try tucking a cushion or a rolled up towel into the nape of your neck. If you have been used to wearing a neck support for a long time, then by now the muscles of your neck will be weak and possibly wasted. Good posture will help these muscles to begin to work for you without the need for such support.

As an additional check on your posture, try this. Stand with your back against a wall and place your hand in the space between your back and the wall at waist level. Now, keeping your shoulders and buttocks firmly against the wall and looking straight ahead, try to reduce the gap by tightening the stomach and buttock muscles. You will find this easier to do if your heels are about 3 inches away from the wall, your feet a little apart and your knees slightly bent. Standing in this position will not only make you aware of the need to tuck in your tummy but will actually relieve a backache. Practise this several times a day.

Developing this habit will help to undo much of the damage caused by slouching and standing in an unbalanced position where the weight is constantly over one leg, and it will help to reduce the stress on the muscles and the joints. To reduce this stress still further, when standing for long periods, try propping one foot up on a step or a small box. Try this with your back against the wall and note how the gap between your back and the wall has virtually disappeared. This position is also recommended to relieve back pain and to reduce tension on the joints and muscles in the lower back.

Getting out of a seat

You can be helped considerably to reduce strain on your whole body by learning to get out of a seat correctly. This is particularly important when rising from a deep armchair or settee. Using your arms to help you, move your body forward to the edge of the seat. Still sitting, place one foot slightly forward of the other and rise, taking all the weight on both feet and legs. Initially you may find it helpful to rest your hands on your knees to give a sense of added security. After some practice you will probably find you can manage without using your hands. Once you are on your feet, pause a moment and straighten up before attempting to move forward.

Lifting

I do not propose to make any recommendations about lifting except to suggest that you seek guidance from a physiotherapist or occupational therapist who will check that you are lifting correctly.

Sleeping

It is just as important to think about your sleeping posture. Night-time is often difficult for people with pain and you may be helped considerably by starting off the night in a posture that is suitable for your condition. If your problem involves neck and head pain, then preferably you should not use high pillows which raise the head and put a strain on the muscles at the back of the neck. Personally I find that using a Japanese-type neck pillow, shaped rather like a dog's bone, is very comfortable both in bed and also sitting in an armchair.

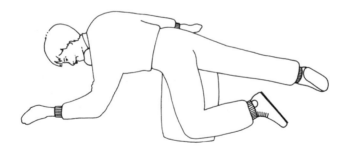

People with back or leg problems can be helped by lying on one side with the upper leg drawn up at the knee and supported by a pillow (see above).

Your weight

Excess weight can add to the burden that the body has to carry, placing strain on joints and muscles and adversely influencing posture. If you are overweight, then, as part of your strategy for managing your pain, you should combine your exercises with a sensible reducing diet. Your doctor can advise on the correct foods for you, but the basic principle to follow is: *eat less and exercise more!*

Keeping fit

As my problem is progressive I have to adapt constantly to changes in my physical capacity as muscles in different parts of my body develop weakness. I have learned that it is important always to work on strengthening the strongest parts of my body whilst at the same time working on the weaker parts to prevent wastage. My walking has become seriously affected during the last two years and I have been concerned to ensure that my leg muscles are still exercised and the rest of my body is kept in good condition.

My wife and I have rediscovered the fun of cycling and the sheer pleasure of working out at a fitness centre. Fitness and leisure centres can be found in any part of the country and abroad. They are not just there for the young and fit. On the contrary I have presented myself on a number of occasions on a pair of crutches or in a wheelchair and been welcomed and treated just the same as any other member of the public. After explaining my particular problems to the staff I have had a programme tailor-made to suit my particular needs. I enjoy the exercise machines, designed to exercise specific muscle groups, and I am able to follow a progressive programme knowing that my body is fully supported. It costs no more than a session at the swimming baths – or a couple of lottery tickets! I certainly feel the benefit physically and a visit there often helps me to get over a set-back. I often arrive in a very sorry state but leave feeling on top of the world. An added bonus of dealing with a set-back in this way is that I have continued to make normal social contact with fit people. It is far better than retreating into the role of 'sick' person.

5

Take Control of your Pain –
Take Control of your Life

John, aged 62, had back and chest pains for more than 10 years. He was a trained engineer but before entering the pain management course he had been unable to work for over two years. He described himself as a 'zombie', hooked on pain-killers. 'If a drug company made it, then I was on it. . . . I have lost count of the number of painkillers I was on each day.' His reaction to all aspects of learning about pain, exercise and relaxation was, to say the least, antagonistic. 'I thought I was going to get proper medical treatment – if all these doctors have not been able to fix me then I am sure you can't. Nobody is going to get into my mind.'

It took two weeks for John to adapt his attitude and during this time he admits he was disruptive in the group. He showed his feelings by walking out and banging doors, lighting up cigarettes during relaxation periods and making disparaging comments. However, the group leaders and members intervened and told him in no uncertain terms that he could think and feel as he wished but in the group his behaviour was not acceptable. However, although outwardly resistant, John had been listening and quietly, on his own, had tried out some of the techniques presented on the course, with pleasing results. At the end of two weeks John showed his courage when he apologized to everyone concerned about his behaviour and started to co-operate fully.

Three years later he proudly acknowledges that '. . . the course changed me from a zombie to a human being. The family are delighted that I am enjoying life again. I realize now that I was really at war with myself.' Because I can relax and am aware of the difference between tension and relaxation, I know exactly which part of my body is not at ease and I can take steps to remedy this immediately – sometimes, simply by pausing for a moment and getting my breathing right. . . . I have taken no painkillers of any kind during the past two-and-a-half years.'

John's story is typical of those who have been locked in pain for a long time. Many patients who are advised to learn relaxation or stress management techniques initially suspect that this is another example of the professionals giving up on treatment or on finding the real cause of the pain, or they may worry that the doctors have found something sinister which they are unwilling to tell them. They may even interpret what the doctors say as meaning that the problem is all in the mind and the pain is imagined. These feelings may have crossed your own mind, especially if you have been from one medical practitioner to another seeking out a cure and receiving different explanations or treatment for your pain, with little lasting relief. If the doctors had found anything sinister, you can be sure that treatment would have been decisive and swift.

Like John, you may take a great deal of convincing that it is possible to give up the belief that someone, somewhere has the precise cure which has so far eluded you and accept that just by learning the skill of relaxation life can take on a new meaning as you experience once more the sensation of being in control.

Taking control

Most of us have been brought up to believe that medical treatment is a process during which we have something 'done to us'. We are used to feeding our symptoms to our doctor and in return being given a prescription which, most of the time, produces satisfactory results. We still cling to the belief that when we see a professional we hand over our problem and expect it to be sorted out. Difficulties arise when we get a condition which will not go away in spite of all the best efforts of the professionals. Naturally, people who have chronic pain often feel let down and fear that if the professionals cannot help them they must be beyond help. At this point it can rightly be said that the patient feels the whole situation seems out of control. It appears that the pain will never go away. Not only do you have the physical pain but, with it, feelings of depression, anger and isolation. This can be really frightening. As a result, you are adding an additional severe stress to that produced by the pain and this increases the feeling of being out of control.

Your chronic pain problem may also increase, exacting a further physical and emotional toll. A vicious self-feeding, self-perpetuating cycle of pain, stress, tension, fear, anxiety, more pain, more stress, and so on, is well and truly established. For example, tension resulting from this not-so-merry-go-round may produce circulation problems arising from decreased blood flow. Adrenalin and other hormones released into the bloodstream can constrict blood vessels so that the blood flows away from your extremities and you will notice that your muscles contract and your hands and feet become cold. You may also have noticed that your sweat level increases so that your skin feels cold and clammy. Digestive problems can arise from increased stomach acidity which in turn may contribute to the development of an ulcer. The constant bracing of shoulder, head and neck muscles, tensed against the pain, can lead to headaches or facial pain. Tension produces an increase in the heart rate and you may have been aware of palpitations and pounding in your chest. You may also have noticed that your breathing is shallow, that you gulp down air periodically, and that your chest muscles are tight.

A disturbed sleep pattern is another major problem for the chronic pain sufferer. Many people say that they have disturbed nights because of pain and as a result feel exhausted and find an overwhelming desire to sleep during the day. The sleep disturbance usually comes about as a result of tension being present in the body at the time of going to sleep. An exhausted, tense body offers fertile ground for pain to grow and to be reinforced by a stream of negative thoughts and images which many pain patients claim is their biggest obstacle to sound sleep.

If you recognize these symptoms it is little wonder you feel out of control. But there is a way out!

Learning to relax effectively

Learning to relax effectively is going to help you in the same way that it has helped John and many thousands of other people who share your problems. Any effective relaxation strategy should also include techniques for developing positive thought patterns and stopping the flow of destructive, anxiety-provoking, tension-producing, negative thought. It is important only to have those thoughts in your mind that you wish to be there. Learning good relaxation techniques to use before settling down for the night and during the disturbed spells is essential.

Relaxation does not mean lounging, reclining, sleeping, watching TV or reading. It is a special skill which we all possess as children and which most of us forget in adult life. However, it can be re-learned if you follow some simple instructions which are designed to give you confidence and help you to get back into control.

Relaxation is a process during which you will allow all the tension to move away from every muscle and organ of your body. During the process of deep relaxation the blood will flow more freely throughout your whole system. Waste products will drain freely, thus decreasing any toxicity within you. Certain forms of relaxation lower the blood pressure and all forms of relaxation produce feelings of calmness and well-being. What is really important to the pain sufferer is that the chemicals (endorphins) responsible for closing the gates to your pain will be produced more freely during relaxation.

It is preferable to have the guidance of someone experienced in teaching methods of relaxation but do not be put off if you do not have access to someone who specializes in this form of teaching. It is a skill which is possible to learn by means of a book and perhaps with the aid of a relaxation cassette tape.

The relaxation programmes begin by presenting straightforward physical methods of achieving the relaxed state, concentrating on breathing techniques, and tightening and relaxing groups of muscles in turn so that you can experience for yourself the difference between relaxation and tension. These methods are often sufficient for pain sufferers to gain control once more of things that are happening inside their own bodies and as a result they find they benefit by having less pain and they develop confidence to use their bodies more freely.

Some people find that physical methods alone are not sufficient so I have included a number of ways in which you will be invited to use your imagination and to recall positive experiences in your life in order to develop your relaxation skills. This process is often called self-hypnosis. Do not be put off by this term – again, it is a label used mainly by psychotherapists to describe a particular form of psycho-logical treatment. Unfortunately, most of us associate the word 'hypnosis' with stage and TV entertainments where people are encouraged to make an exhibition of themselves for the pleasure of the audience. What you see on stage is entirely different from the therapeutic use of one of the most powerful forms of treatment available. A form of hypnosis was used by the ancient Greeks in order to induce a calm relaxed state which would allow the body to heal itself without the need for any other form of intervention.

Hypnotherapy, and particularly the practice of self-hypnosis, enables people to develop and enhance their own ability to control what is going on in their minds and bodies. A visit to a qualified and experienced hypnotherapist is an enjoyable, civilized experience, where every concern is shown for the patient's comfort. Just think how pleasant it must be to be treated without the intervention of drugs, needles, or knives! So do not let the word 'hypnosis' frighten you. If you visit a hypnotherapist for any problem, but particularly for the management of chronic pain, you will be taught methods of self-hypnosis because in the long-term this tuition will be the most beneficial.

All I am asking you to do is to try for yourself the various relaxation techniques described so that you can decide for yourself which help you most.

Preparing yourself for relaxation

It is necessary to withdraw from the family, the telephone, and other intrusions to your peace whilst you are learning. People suffering pain or anxiety from whatever cause will benefit from following this programme. It is important that you set aside two or three half-hour periods a day so that you can experience for yourself the difference between tension and relaxation and eventually reach a stage where you are able to switch on relaxation automatically. If this seems very demanding, think of the time you have spent lying down or lounging around locked in negative thought and pain for many hours each day. This is surely a much more positive way to spend time.

It would be helpful to get someone to read through the instructions for you to follow or alternatively record them on cassette so that they can be used at any time of the day – or night. Make sure that all relaxation exercises are done in a warm room and wear comfortable, loose clothing and socks. If you wish, cover yourself with a blanket or duvet. There is a tendency for the body to cool during deep relaxation.

Relaxation programme

Getting started

Basic to all relaxation skills is breathing. People who are in pain or who are anxious or tense, breathe shallowly. Deep breathing is one of the easiest ways to release tension in the body. You were probably taught at some time in your life to 'breathe deeply and throw your chest out'. If you try this you will experience tightness in the muscles across your chest. This form of breathing is not relaxing. In fact, if you can become aware of your breathing during your pain attack or an anxiety attack, or if you remember a time when you were frightened, you will notice that tightness is the characteristic breathing response in these situations. People who have pain and who breathe this way are actually making their situation worse by creating tense muscles and disturbing the oxygen supply to the rest of the body. Correct diaphragmatic breathing can help to release tension, reduce anxiety and control fear and it provides the means to step out of the vicious circle. It can be practised anywhere, any time, alone or in the company of others, whatever you are doing, walking, sitting, lying down – in fact in any situation where you feel the need to relieve tension and pain.

Initially you may feel that you are achieving very little or that the exercises are not helping you – but persevere, make them a part of your daily routine and eventually they will help you to ease your stress and discomfort. Some people experience a dramatic improvement simply because of the increased oxygen supply and the release from tension and they are tempted to think they have been 'cured'. But this is dangerous thinking! The exercises must be done *regularly* and be incorporated into your normal daily activities – just like cleaning your teeth.

When first learning the technique, it is best to lie down on your back with your legs straight in front with your feet a comfortable distance apart or with knees bent and feet flat on the floor. To become aware of your breathing, place one hand on your chest and one on your diaphragm, just below the centre of the rib-cage. Breathe in slowly and easily through the nostrils allowing the air to move through the chest and into your stomach. As the breath reaches your stomach, push your diaphragm upwards towards the ceiling allowing this hand to rise higher than the hand on your chest. Hold for a second then allow the breath to pass out through the chest and nostrils. As you breathe out, feel all your muscles let go of tension. Continue to breathe in this way for several minutes. You may find this process difficult at first but it is worth persevering and your body will let you know when you are comfortable with this method of breathing.

Variation 1

A variation of this technique which some people find more helpful is to lie down as before and, as you breathe out, place both hands on the diaphragm so that the tips of your fingers of each hand are just touching. When you breathe in, push the diaphragm upwards, your fingers should part. When you breathe out, allow the diaphragm to fall and your fingers should touch again. As with the first method, practise this for several minutes. Learn to monitor your breathing constantly throughout the day. It is possible to keep one small part of your mind focused on your breathing at all times so that you can become aware of any changes instantly and correct your breathing pattern. Each time you practise relaxing this way it will become easier. As your skill develops, practise when you are standing, sitting, or doing jobs around the house.

The aim of this method and all the other methods which I am describing, is to reduce the resting tension in the muscles. Although at times you may think you are relaxed, your muscles may still be tensed. It is important to develop an awareness of when you are tense and when you are relaxed and to be able to spot the increase of tension early thereby preventing muscle tension from developing.

Variation 2

Many people, including myself, find this next variation particularly useful in that it helps to develop an awareness of diaphragmatic breathing, to make the breathing deeper and to bring quick relief from back pain. Place a thin pillow or cushion on the floor and lie face down with the pillow under the diaphragm, and the head turned to one side. Arms should lie comfortably along the side of the body. As you inhale, feel your abdomen pressing against the cushion. As you slowly exhale, feel the abdominal muscles relaxing. Spend a few minutes in this position. Some people find it so

61

comfortable that they drift into a relaxed sleep but this is not important as the main purpose of the exercise is to become aware of diaphragmatic movement. As you become comfortable with deep breathing exercises you can move on to a technique called Progressive Muscle Relaxation, developed by Jacobson in the 1930s. This technique is designed to eliminate muscle tension by contracting the various groups of muscles in the body and releasing the tension slowly. It is very effective in helping people to learn about muscle tension and to be aware of the sharp contrast between tense muscles and relaxed muscles. Many people spend the day in a tensed state with clenched teeth or fists or shoulders and do not even realize it until bed-time when a headache or neck and shoulder pain results. Unawareness of tension in the muscles can lead to muscle fatigue, poor circulation, cramps and stiffness and an exacerbation of your pain problem. It is the tension in the muscles which makes them more prone to spasm. If you have any particularly painful area, avoid over-tensing this and the muscles surrounding it. Take this exercise slowly at first. Do not strain. You may experience cramp but it will go away as you release the tension.

Instructions for progressive muscle relaxation

Exercise 1
Sit in a fully supported position in a chair or lie down on your back on the floor. Become aware of your breathing for a minute or two, feeling the INbreath flowing into the diaphragm and allowing the breathing rhythm to become easy and comfortable. If you find the breathing difficult at this stage it is probably because you are trying too hard. When your breathing is steady and comfortable focus your attention on the arms. Lift them slightly, extend them, clench the fists as hard as you can. Now, hold the tension in your fists . . . and your arms, . . . breathe in and slowly count up to 5 . . . then let the tension go, breathing out as you do so and let the arms fall back into the resting position. Feel the muscles go limp. Feel the increased bloodflow into the hands and fingers. Take note of the contrast between the muscles as they were when tense and the way they are when relaxed.

Repeat this exercise 3 times.

Exercise 2

Take a deep breath, hold it. Now raise the shoulders towards the ears at the same time pulling the head down towards the shoulders. Hold the breath and the tension for a count of 5 then release the breath and the tension and allow the shoulders to relax.
   Repeat 3 times.

Exercise 3

Take a deep breath into the chest, hold it for a count of 5 whilst tensing the muscles in the chest area, then let go the breath and the tension, allowing all the muscles to relax completely.
   Repeat this 3 times.

Now, spend several moments restoring the breathing into the diaphragm and proceed to the next exercise when you feel comfortable.

Exercise 4

If you are lying down, just bend the knees slightly. Tighten up the muscles around the abdomen and pelvic area. Breathe in, hold the breath and the tension for a count of 5 then let go the breath and the tension.
   Repeat 3 times.

This is a good stage to pause for a while and to take note of what is happening in your body. You should be feeling an increased blood flow and perhaps an increase in warmth around the neck, the hands and the arms. This is the time to think about your breathing. If you find that it has a tendency to get shallow, make sure you are not continuing to hold your breath during the relaxation phase of the exercise. If this is happening then take time between each phase to restore your diaphragmatic breathing.

Exercise 5

Tighten the muscles of your buttocks as hard as you can, take a deep breath and hold the tension and the breath for a count of 5. Let go the tension and the breath, allowing the muscles to relax completely.
   Repeat 3 times.

Exercise 6

Tighten the muscles of the thighs as hard as you can. Take a deep breath, hold the tension and the breath for a count of 5. Let go the tension and the breath, letting the muscles relax completely.

Repeat 3 times.

Exercise 7

With feet together and legs stretched out in front of you, tighten the muscles of your feet and calves by pointing your toes away from you as hard as you can. Take a deep breath, hold the tension and the breath for a count of 5. Now let go the tension and the breath allowing the muscles relax completely. To complete this exercise stretch the legs again in front of you, tighten the muscles of your feet and calves by pointing your toes towards you as hard as you can. Take a deep breath, hold the tension and the breath for a count of 5. Now, let go the tension and the breath, allowing the muscles to relax completely.

Repeat 3 times.

Now establish your breathing into your diaphragm and rest quietly. Experience the feeling of complete relaxation throughout your whole body.

Exercise 8

This final exercise is particularly good for people with head, face and neck pains where a build up of tension can make the problem seem so much worse.

Try not to be self-conscious about this one and set out to enjoy it. If you feel like laughing do so because laughter helps to reduce tension in a way that no other exercise can.

Start by tightening the muscles in the jaw and neck area. Stretch the mouth to make a narrow grinning expression on your face at the same time stick out your tongue as far as it will go, screw up the eyes, take a deep breath, hold the tension, count up to 5 and then let go the tension and the breath and relax completely.

Repeat 3 times.

Now, open the eyes wide and look towards the ceiling, open the mouth wide and allow the jaw to drop. Take a deep breath, hold the position to a count of 5 and then let go the breath, close the mouth and eyes and relax.

Remain in your relaxed position and if you wish you can continue with the next phase of learning the relaxation response.

Make this physical form of relaxation part of your daily routine. This will help you keep physically toned up, relaxed, and give you a warm feeling which can stay with you for most of the day.

Instructions for relaxation

Now that you have begun to be aware of the difference between tension and relaxation and to feel the changes taking place in your body as the blood flows freely to every part of it, you will be learning unconsciously (if not already consciously) that you can, in fact, change the way your body feels. Now is the time to build on this experience and to start learning that you can produce the same good feelings by using thought processes only.

So that these instructions for relaxation techniques can be read out or recorded in the most helpful way, I have marked pauses by a series of dots (. . . .) each dot roughly representing one second. It is important that the person reading or making a recording is as relaxed as possible.

Now, sit in a fully supported position in a chair or, if preferred, lie down, with your eyes closed. Establish your breathing into your diaphragm. . . . . remember .. there is no rush at all about these exercises. [Pause for about 30 seconds to allow the breathing pattern to be established.]

Try not to be distracted by noises inside or outside the room . . . . just become aware of them for a moment. . . . . . then let them go . . . . they are not important . . . . .

It is important that no worrying thoughts remain in your mind during the exercise. . If they occur just let them go through your mind and out again. . . . . Some people find that it helps to use a word at this stage to help the relaxation process to get established quickly and to exclude sounds and thoughts which can intrude . . . . . . It is very difficult to block out all thought . . . .therefore it is

65

helpful to use a word like CALM or the name of a colour which has a relaxing connotation such as BLUE . . . .

Think of the word each time you breathe out. . . . Slow down your breathing. . . . . and try to make each OUTbreath longer than the INbreath. . . . . Establish your own slow . . rhythmic . . pace . . . . remembering that this is your own special time. . . to enjoy.

As your relaxation deepens, become aware . . . of your arms . . .your hands . . . your fingers. Let go mentally of any tension that may be there . . . . . you don't need to do anything . . . . just think of any tension moving away from this part of your body. . . . . Be aware of the way your arms and your hands feel . . . . some people feel heaviness. . . . some feel a tingling sensation . . . . some feel the warmth of deepening relaxation . . . . . . Enjoy this feeling for a few moments as you continue to breathe slowly . . . . and rhythmically. . .

Now turn your attention to your shoulders and the back of your neck . . and let go all the tension in that area . . . .

Now be aware of your head, particularly the area round your eyes . . . . it is important to let ALL the tension go around your eyes . . . . . and the muscles of your face . . . . . let the tension go from there . . . .

Become aware of any tension around your jaw . . . . . If your teeth are clenched tightly together . . . . just let them part slightly . . . . . and rest your tongue lightly behind your lower teeth . . . . .

Now be aware of the muscles of your chest . . . . . let the tension go from there . . . . . and the muscles of your stomach . . . . . . and your pelvis . . . . and your lower back . . . . let all the tension move away from this area . . . . . . Be aware of your feelings of deepening relaxation in this part of your body. . . . . . and enjoy them . . . .

Be aware now of your buttocks. . . and your thighs . . . . these areas can get very tense whether you are sitting or standing . . . . . just let ALL the tension go . . . .

Now your legs . . . your ankles . . . . . your feet. . . and your toes . . . Let all remaining tension flow from your body. . . . . Imagine it flowing out through the ends of your toes. . . . . . .

If you want to use this relaxation programme as a prelude to sleep then insert the following words at this point:

..... and continuing to breathe deeply, just drift into a relaxed sleep .... a sleep from which you will awake refreshed..... calm .... and with a feeling of optimism about the new day ahead ...

Lie for the next two or three minutes enjoying the feeling of deep relaxation ....
[Allow a few minutes to elapse.]

And now, slowly become aware of your body........ a relaxed body ..... Slowly move your fingers and toes ..... allowing the feeling to come back into your hands and feet ..... and, keeping that feeling of relaxation, allow your eyes to open. Don't rush to get up.

You may not find much difference at first but it is important that you go through the process at least once a day until your mind and your body establish the habit of deep relaxation. Above all, do not worry that you are failing. Some days you may find the whole process easy and comfortable; other days you may find relaxation eludes you. This is normal so don't give up! As you get more skilled you will find that establishing diaphragmatic breathing and using the word you have chosen will be sufficient to induce a very deep level of relaxation throughout the whole body. This is what you are aiming for.

If you still have any doubts that you, yourself can produce beneficial changes in your body and in the way you feel, just close your eyes for a moment, breathe into your diaphragm, slowly .... and easily .... and bring into your mind a memory of a time when things were very good for you, perhaps the proudest moment of your life, a day when everything went right and you felt at your best. Everyone has such a moment. Allow a picture of that time to emerge .... see it .... feel it .... hear it ..... you may even smell it – but above all, enjoy it. Notice how you feel inside.

By way of contrast, close your eyes, breathe deeply into your diaphragm and think for a moment of your pain and discomfort. Notice how you feel ... and switch as quickly as you can to the pleasant memory you have just had and enjoy it to the full once more. Again, notice how you feel – and remember that good feeling, particularly the changes that have taken place in your body. If you wish at this point, you can continue with your eyes closed, enjoying this memory and perhaps even stay in a relaxed comfortable state for a few minutes.

I use the above exercise frequently when working with groups of people to help them become aware of just how powerful their own minds are in producing changes and to demonstrate yet another way into becoming deeply relaxed. Without exception, the group members find this exercise particularly useful and refreshing.

The biofeedback monitor

If you go to hospital for treatment you may be introduced to a biofeedback machine. Biofeedback is used to train people to relax tension in various parts of their bodies. Electrodes are used to connect various parts of your body to the machine to give feedback about how tensed or relaxed your muscles are, how cold your hands may be, how much you sweat, and how fast your heart beats, providing measurements which indicate your degree of relaxation. You may be asked to sit and observe the movement of a needle on a dial or listen to a tone as you practise various ways of relaxing. Obviously, these machines are very expensive for use at home but they are an invaluable tool for measuring tension and for demonstrating the part that you the individual plays in bringing about changes in your own body. Some people find this a more acceptable way of learning control than the other methods I have outlined. Fortunately a simple, effective machine for home use is available at an affordable price from a well-known national electronic equipment chainstore. It works by the attachment of pads to the ends of two fingers and measures quite simply the amount of sweat being produced on the surface of your skin. The more tense you are, the more sweat is produced. A high-pitched sound clearly demonstrates a high degree of tension within the body. As you become more relaxed the sound diminishes in intensity and it is possible to achieve a state of relaxation which is sufficiently deep to stop the sound altogether. Whilst attached to this machine, it is useful to experiment by tensing one or more groups of muscles in turn and observe the changes. A number of patients I have worked with have experimented by thinking of things which cause them discomfort or tension and have learned very quickly just how sensitive the machine can be to these unpleasant thoughts that cause changes in the body. The machine itself is merely a measuring tool – it does not do anything to the body, it merely records information and feeds it back to you.

The part that memory and imagination can play in making you feel more comfortable

If you have had your pain for a long time it may seem as though nothing pleasant ever happens, but this is not so! Probably for 90% of your life things have gone well but unfortunately this problem that you have is over-shadowing all the good things that have ever happened to you. During your life you have faced and solved many problems and as a result you have learned a great deal. You have also had many pleasurable experiences. The wonderful thing is that the memories related to these are still with you but because of your present difficulties they have been pushed deep inside you. During relaxation it is possible to get in touch with these positive aspects of your life, recalling in detail all the events and the good feelings attached to them. It is rather like helping you to look back through a photograph album and each picture can stimulate your mind to produce a whole flood of memories that you thought were long forgotten. In deep relaxation when these memories are stimulated you can begin to feel now exactly as you did when the events first happened. The return of these positive feelings not only has a beneficial effect on your mind, helping you to feel better, but, at the same time, physiological changes take place so that the body is stimulated to work more efficiently generally so that blood flow increases, more endorphins are produced and waste products are eliminated more easily.

You may have heard or read about 'imagery and visualization' and this really means using your imagination to reduce the effects of illness and discomfort. Your imagination is very powerful and, properly used, can be effective in stimulating the body to heal itself and to relieve pain. It is possible to learn how to use your imagination for your own benefit and most people very soon develop the skill. Again, it is useful to have the instructions read to you, or taped whilst you are learning.

Try this:

Sit well supported in a chair, if necessary with your back, neck and head supported by pillows. If you wish you may lie down. The choice is yours, whichever is more comfortable. Make sure you are warm and go into a state of relaxation just as you did for relaxation by thought processes only ......(as described on p. 65) and continue as follows:

Now that your relaxation has been established and you have removed all the tension from your body, remember a time when you experienced the warmth of the sun on your back. Remember a time – it may be many years ago, it may be quite recently – when you had an experience, (a pleasant experience; a comfortable experience) perhaps an occasion when you enjoyed the warmth of the sun in the company of other people. You may have enjoyed a holiday and recall the sights, the sounds, and smells of that holiday. Remember the things that made you laugh. Remember .... how freely you moved .... and how good you felt .... Feel the warmth and comfort spreading through the whole of your body. Now just imagine the sun moving to focus its rays on that particular part of you which causes discomfort ...... Experience the warmth in that area ..... and the way the warmth changes the way it feels. Imagine that the warmth of the sun can stay there bringing feelings of comfort and ease ..... knowing that when this exercise is over these pleasant feelings can remain with you .... and you will be able to get back to this pleasant state any time you wish ......

Now, rest quietly for a few minutes enjoying this experience.....
[Allow 2 or 3 minutes to elapse before continuing.]

And, now, gradually become aware of your body and in your own good time knowing that you can carry these good feelings with you, and feeling refreshed, begin to move your fingers and gradually awake completely.

In addition to using memory to stimulate your imagination, you can choose anything you like to symbolize your pain. It can be shape, size, colour, a word, an animal or bird. The principle is the same – finding a means of changing the symbol you have chosen to represent your pain into something more tolerable and more pleasant, for example, changing a dark colour to a light colour or a crow into a bird of paradise!

Switch off

Another way to use your imagination involves going into deep relaxation using deep breathing combined with one of the methods already described and then following these instructions:

You are probably aware ...... that everything that goes on inside your body is controlled or monitored by some part of the brain. It is your brain which is receiving messages from all parts of your body .... some of them pleasant .... some not so pleasant.. some positively frightening .....As you have become progressively more skilled in relaxation ....and have begun to learn .... that *you* yourself .... have control over processes which previously you believed were beyond your control .... then now is the time to take another step in learning.... how to change .. the way your body feels.........

As you go deeper into relaxation ......imagine that you have the special ability to enter your own head to wander around .... and explore what is going on.... Just imagine .. you can find that part of the brain which is linked to that particular part of your body which is causing you concern... Look around to see if you can find the switch that connects the two together... It may be that it is on a control panel, perhaps even labelled ..... Before you reach out and press the switch, just think for a moment 'Is this switch going to .....turn down the volume ... or might it even .... change ...the unpleasant sensation .. to a pleasant feeling .. an enjoyable feeling ....or perhaps that switch might even ... switch off the pain altogether'. Now, reach out and press the switch.

Enjoy the experience of deep relaxation combined with a feeling of pleasure and comfort resulting from the knowledge that *you* have the ability to find the means of producing positive changes. And now .. rest quietly for a few minutes. [Allow two or three minutes to pass before going on.]

And now, still feeling comfortable, become aware of where you are, become aware of your body. Move your fingers and toes and, when you are ready, feeling fully alert, open your eyes and be wide awake.

A couple of years ago I was working with a group of patients using this particular method. Jean, a young lady of 19 who had severe arthritis in her spine, when asked to explore and find the switch suddenly burst out laughing, saying she knew exactly where she was. 'I'm in the Thunderbirds control room. I can see Brains in front of the control panel. Brains is going to press my switch . . . and Brains is going to turn off my pain.' The method certainly worked for Jean and she often used her relaxation time to activate the switch with the aid of 'Brains'.

Imagination works in different ways for different people, personally when relaxing and using visualization, the switch method is not so effective for me. I prefer to work in colour, changing from dark to light. You may find it helps to explore the most effective way to use your imagination, by trying each one in turn. Although you may not feel your pain directly influenced on any one occasion, you will probably find that going through the process will progressively enable you to see that over a period you are experiencing less pain, with less frequency and that your ability to recover from 'flare-ups' or set-backs, is increased. You may also find that you become more optimistic, more active, less anxious or depressed.

This improvement can be further reinforced by the following set of instructions. They are particularly designed to produce feelings of hope and to encourage the practitioner to feel more alert and active.

Sit with your back, head and neck well-supported.....or lie down if your prefer... for the next few moments concentrate on your breathing, breathing into your diaphragm, making your ouтbreath longer than your INbreath .... and you slow down your breathing, making it deeper ... allow your relaxation to become deeper. What you are aiming for is a state of relaxation which enables you to let go all tension from your body, allowing it to move away from ....your head .... your eyes ... around your jaw ... your neck ... your shoulders .... your arms ... and hands. Allow the tension to move away from your back.... your chest ... your stomach ... your pelvic area and buttocks ... your thighs ... your legs .. your ankles .... and your feet. Experience this relaxation for a few moments..... knowing that while your body is completely relaxed, your mind is clear and sharp.

By now you have lived through many seasons and you know that every season is different. I have no doubt that in the past you have experienced many things some of them you may recall easily – others may seem to be lost in the mists of time. You may not have realized it but these memories, these important memories, can be of use to you in your present difficulties. You can probably remember a summer ... a warm summer ... a happy summer, a summer when .. you moved around freely, enjoying the sun on your face, in the company of good friends, the pleasure of moving without effort. You may have had many summers like this ... in fact, for a long time you probably remember feeling exactly like this whatever the season of the year. However, that summer season may have changed for you so that you experienced the cold chill of autumn ... the growing darkness ... and perhaps even the bitter cold as winter approached. It may be that ... sensitive to this change ... you wrapped yourself around for protection, just as the caterpillar protects himself from the frost of autumn and winter by enveloping himself in a chrysalis to survive the bitter chill, the darkness and discomfort of winter....

But you know, as I know ..... that winter is always followed by *spring*! and that spring brings a re-awakening .....the chrysalis opens in the warmth of the sun to allow the beautiful butterfly to emerge into the light... full of energy ... full of life...ready to enjoy again the pleasure of the Summer ... the pleasure of moving without effort .. As you remember these things you can resolve to take these good feelings with you as you begin ... once more ... enjoy an activity ...which you have not done for some time. It may simply be a walk in the park... or by a river, with the sunlight sparkling on it .... listening to the sound of the birds ... looking up to the sky to see the movement of soft, white clouds ... Enjoy this scene, and increasingly ... feel more energetic ... more hopeful ... and more able to experience the pleasure of living your life to the full.

Getting back to sleep

You may find it difficult to get off to sleep, wake in the night, or find you are too sleepy to get up in the morning and doze at intervals during the day. This disturbed sleep pattern is common. Several factors are responsible. The severity of the pain may prevent you from getting off to sleep. Discomfort arising from lying down in one position for too long may wake you up, tension which has built up throughout the day can be released from knotted, tight muscles during the night and this can cause restlessness and even pain.

Getting into bed or waking in the night can often be the signals for a negative stream of thoughts about your health and your seemingly hopeless situation to be switched on – and as you know, these can produce tension and increase your pain. Frustration and anger at your inability to sleep can produce further tension.

In this situation sleeplessness can become a habit. It is likely that you go to bed expecting to have difficulty getting off to sleep and believing firmly that you will wake up sometime in the night – because you always do. These expectations can be worrying and it is quite likely that you will live up to them having programmed yourself to a pattern of behaviour which is unhelpful to your attempts to manage your pain and your life.

NOW is the time to work on changing this unhelpful pattern. Fortunately, if you choose to develop good pain management techniques of exercise and increased activity combined with regular relaxation sessions many of your sleep problems will ease and may even disappear altogether.

To capitalize on this improvement, consider changing other aspects of your behaviour:

1. Get up at a fixed time each morning, preferably with the family who may be going off to school or work. If you live alone, then fix a time no later than 8.30.

2. If you find yourself beginning to doze during the day, get up and go out for a walk or do something absorbing and do some exercise. Set yourself times for complete relaxation using one of the methods I have described. Relaxation does not mean nodding off!

3. Avoid at all costs sitting watching television for long periods, and – if you have got into the habit of watching throughout the day and evening, then think about switching off. Much of TV viewing is a habit and one which can keep you in a sitting position for long periods thereby increasing the likelihood of pain. TV is far from relaxing – it is exhausting.

Even a short programme can induce numerous physiological

changes as a whole range of emotions is rapidly experienced – sadness, anger, fear, sexual tension, and as a result chemicals are released into the bloodstream for no useful purpose at all! The real purpose of these chemicals is to enable us to meet challenges and cope with danger and to equip us for normal everyday activities. When you cope with the challenges in reality, the flow ceases and you then relax naturally. However, if the release is provoked by second-hand experience as when watching a TV programme, then you are left with a surfeit of substances in the bloodstream which feed your tension and, consequently, your pain.

So limit your viewing, especially news bulletins 'on the hour every hour'. Ration yourself to one news bulletin a day. The world will carry on just the same without you worrying about how to put it right. You have got quite enough problems of your own to cope with and do not need to be fed with endless tales of disaster and catastrophe presented in gory detail. Above all, avoid getting embroiled emotionally in the endless audience participation arguments, political or otherwise, which pass for 'entertainment'. They only increase tension.

4. Change your bedtime routine – if you are tired before your 'usual' bedtime then go to bed then – don't wait up. Get used to switching off TV putting down your book or newspaper and avoid getting into heated discussions with other members of the household at least one hour before bedtime. Wind down slowly. Take yourself off for a warm bath then have a warm drink. Take your time and enjoy it. Make sure your bedroom and your bed are warm and if you have a cassette player, put on a relaxation tape or soft music and switch off the light. Make this a habit following the same sequence each night. As you rest your head on the pillow and listen to your tape, begin to breathe into your diaphragm. The aim is to release, through your breathing and relaxation, all the resting tension in your muscles. Let thoughts just drift through your head but don't hold on to them. Try taking yourself in your imagination to a warm comfortable place.

5. Learn to deal with negative thoughts. You only want things in your mind which *you* put there. If you are troubled by them try this; tense yourself completely, breathe in deeply, hold your breath for five seconds and mentally shout 'STOP' as loud as you can. Let go

your breath, let go all the tension in your muscles and relax completely.

6. If you wake in the night learn to accept your sleeplessness without getting upset at yourself or your situation. Remember negative thoughts are unhelpful – make sure you are warm and comfortable and try your relaxation tape. If you have already had up to five hours sleep then try getting up and moving around. Get dressed, exercise, or go for a walk and get on with your day. It is quite possible you have had enough sleep, particularly if you have not been active during the day.

Calming and restoring balance

By now you will have begun to appreciate that physical and emotional well-being are indivisible. If you have already begun to exercise you will have experienced the benefits of reduced tension and increased relaxation.

It is quite possible that if you have had pain for a long time you have developed a stoop or a tilt to the side. This tendency to get out of balance is more common as we get older and has a lot to do with habits we have developed over the years. You may have noticed that anyone used to carrying a shoulder bag, unconsciously holds one shoulder noticeably higher than the other, even when the bag isn't on it. When working with self-help groups I have found that it is almost impossible to persuade people that they would be more comfortable, and their pain less, if they tried to get out of this habit. Someone using a walking stick for support may develop tensions on one side of the body and lean to one side as a result. People with pain develop different ways of guarding themselves against the pain. This often means tensing muscles, and over a long period the way you stand, sit or walk is altered in such a way that you find it difficult to maintain a vertical position.

The following exercises are designed to help you feel what it is like to be balanced and comfortable. For many people it provides a breakthrough to understanding that they have complete control over their body and their feelings.

You will find it helpful to have someone read out the instructions.

So that you can be sensitive to adjustments in your stance it is better to do this exercise without shoes, preferably in bare feet, on your exercise mat. If you feel that it would be too uncomfortable to remove your shoes and socks then by all means leave them on and just stand on the floor.

Find enough space to allow you to extend your arms sideways.

1. Now, stand with your feet slightly apart (about 9 inches) with your toes pointing forward, fix your eyes straight ahead on a point on the wall in front of you. You may need to have a chair at the side of you for support.

Standing in this way may feel unnatural if you have adopted a 'splayed' stance for comfort or if you are normally a bit pigeon-toed. It may also feel strange if your body has been out of balance for some time. If at any time during this exercise you feel dizzy or distressed, then sit down for a few moments until you feel you can start again.

Continuing to stand in this way, with your arms hanging loosely by your sides, draw yourself up to your full height – feel as if you have a cord coming out of the top of your head like a puppet. Your head should not tilt backwards or forwards and your chin should be parallel to the floor. Holding your head high, gently relax your shoulders down.

Now direct your breathing into your diaphragm and breathe through the nostrils to a count of 4 in and 4 out. It will help you get the right rhythm by allowing about 2 seconds between counts. After 10 full breaths, breathe normally.

Now, keeping the breathing to a 4-in and 4-out count, raise your arms up on the in breath until they are straight out to the side at shoulder level. On the out breath lower them back down to your sides. Your arms should be relaxed with hands hanging loose. You should feel your in breath gently lift your arms away from your sides. Do not push them up. There should be no tension whatever in your body. All your movements should be timed to your breathing and should be smooth, without any break in the middle. As you gain confidence in movement and balance you can extend the breathing to a count of 4 in and 6 out. Remember the section on diaphragmatic breathing and how the out breath should be longer than the in. This helps breath control and any tendency to 'puffing' in and out. This may be enough for your first attempt.

Some people can find that this exercise is quite an effort for them. However, next time you will find you can repeat the exercise and be ready to go on to the next stage. Whatever kind of exercise you are doing, this is a good one for warming up and cooling down.

Add the following exercises over the next two sessions to build up a programme which exercises all parts of the body.

2. After the initial exercises of breathing to a count of 4 in and 4 out, extend this to 4 in and 8 out and at the same time do the arm raising exercise to this count. Again, the aim is to have the arm and breathing synchronized. Repeat twice more.

Then, to a count of 4 in and 8 out, raise the arms to meet above your head and back down to the sides. Repeat twice more.

Now to a count of 6, raise your hands above your head and clasp them together. Hold the clasp – and the breath – for a count of 2, then lower your arms to your sides to a count of 8. Repeat twice more.

To finish, draw your shoulders up to your ear and down again, and generally shake out any parts of the body that feel tight or stretched – hands, arms, legs, feet – until all tension has gone.

3. Place your hands with palms together in front of you in the 'prayer' position. Breathe in to a count of 4, at the same time pressing the palms together, putting tension on the upper arms and shoulders. Hold for 2 or 3 seconds, then breathe out relaxing the hands. Repeat twice more.

Again, place the hands with palms together in 'prayer' position. Now, to a count of 4, breathe in and raise the hands up in front of you, pressing palms together to apply tension, until the arms are straight up above the head. Hold for 2 or 3 seconds then breathe out; still keeping palms together, lower the arms to their starting position. Shake out hands, arms, and legs before repeating twice more.

4. Take up a balanced standing position with your arms relaxed at your sides. Now, looking straight ahead, breathe in to a count of 4 as you *slowly* move your head to the left, half-way between the front and the side. Hold for 2 or 3 seconds, then on the out breath of 4 return the head to the front.

Repeat the same movement again to the left, still breathing in to a count of 4, but this time move your head slightly further round towards the side, *hold*, then breathe out to a count of 4, at the same time moving the head to the front.

Repeat this movement to the same side but this time try to move the head as far as possible. Hold for 2 or 3 seconds, then on the out breath *slowly* take the head round to face the front. Pause and relax as you restore your diaphragmatic breathing.

Repeat the whole sequence moving the head to the right.

At the end of this sequence, remain in the balanced position, enjoying the feeling of warmth resulting from the release of tension in the neck and shoulder muscles. Finish by bringing your shoulders up to your ears, holding for a few seconds, then releasing the tension.

5. The final part of this work-out involves unwinding the top half of the body while putting tension on the legs and hamstrings. Standing in the balanced position with knees locked and arms hanging loosely by the sides, *slowly* lower your chin to your chest. *Very slowly*, carry on lowering the body, one vertabrae at a time, the shoulders, the upper spine; until the top part of the body is hanging over like a rag doll, with arms flopping loosely. There should be absolutely no tension in the body except for the straight legs. The slower you do this exercise the better the effect. When you feel you have been in the hanging position for long enough (this can build up over a period), start to come up, unwinding slowly. Return the same way you went down, i.e. the lowest part comes up first, then the middle, then the upper spine, then the shoulders and last of all the head. In your own time, finish by shrugging the shoulders up to your ears and releasing. Do this several times. If you feel at all uncomfortable or dizzy during this exercise, then stop.

This exercise session should always be followed by a complete relaxation, lying down, covered with a blanket or sleeping bag to maintain body heat.

6

Changing

Changing the script

We have observed earlier how chronic pain changes many aspects of peoples lives, usually for the worse. You yourself will be aware of just how different you feel, look and behave since the onset of your pain. You may have sensed that those around you have changed too and you may not like what you see. This chapter is all about taking responsibility for changing and restructuring every day of your life. By now you should have accepted the advice given in this book that your recovery depends on taking control of various aspects of your life, step by step, and if you have been putting aside part of each day for exercise and practising relaxation, you will now be in a position to appreciate the positive benefits that can be achieved by making small changes in your daily routine.

If, however, you are skimming through the book before you decide to take the plunge and you have not yet been stimulated to put the advice into practice, there is nothing to stop you turning back to the chapters on exercise and relaxation and making the decision *now* to change your daily routine slightly and fit in these new activities. Make this the first step out from your pain. What you do and the order in which you do it is not important. What is important is that *you* decide for yourself that it is time for change. You have spent too long in the pain state and life is too short to spend any more of it in limbo!

You could perhaps 'get by' if you just learn the physical exercises and relaxation skills. They will help you to gain strength and increase your mobility, have more control over your pain and as a result extend your range of activities and increase your enjoyment of life. However, once you see the value of exercise and relaxation you will be ready to move on and accept new challenges and become more adventurous. So, what are these new challenges?

I am interested in taking your rehabilitation even further by helping you to recognize specific areas of your life which would benefit from small changes and to help you identify and remove any obstacles to making the changes.

It can be frightening to think about change as the implications can be enormous. This might be the point when you are faced with resuming responsibility for all sorts of things as you move away from the 'invalid' status where you and your pain have been the central focus of those around you. Well-meaning carers might prefer you to preserve the status quo as you are now part of their new routines and they may fear you may do yourself harm as you move away from what they consider to be a comfortable, well-regulated state. You, though, may recognize the gulf between your present dependent state and the life you would wish to lead and, as you get better, wonder whether you have the courage to give up this protection. This can be a real conflict. However, this cocooned life is unreal and you will have to face up to the fact, as I did, that you are not fully alive.

In the following pages I am going to talk about 'changing the script'. It seems to me that when we get into the chronic pain state and become inactive and dependent on others, it is as if someone has confused us by handing us a script to follow which is completely different to the one which we have been following up to this point in our life. Just imagine TV viewers' confusion watching their favourite 'soap', if one of the characters suddenly took over a different part in the same programme!

This is, in effect, what happens to anyone who has undergone change as a result of pain. Not only do we confuse other people by our change of character but we confuse ourselves and this confusion can be frightening. No doubt, like me, you do not like the changes which have taken place and you recognize that something is wrong, that everything about you is alien. You are not the same person you once were and you wonder where the real you has gone. Fortunately, we can bring back the real you, perhaps even stronger as a result of the experiences you have had and the new learning you have acquired on the journey back.

Certainly, there are risks in meeting the challenge of change – but you have changed before. Sometimes by choice, sometimes you have had change forced upon you – but most of the time you have come through successfully. You do not like what is happening to you now and you want to change for the better. So start now and you will find, as I did, that when your family and friends see the real You begin to emerge, they will lose their fear and earlier reluctance and become eager to encourage you to carry on.

The challenge of change is not so daunting if we think in terms of changing just one small aspect of our own behaviour. In my own case, when I was on the pain management course, I remarked that I would enjoy being able to sit through a meal without having to get up several times to ease my discomfort. Someone suggested that I might try moving to a different seat at the table as that small change might make all the difference. Without really accepting that it would, but because it was such a small change to make, I decided to have a go. It seemed too easy just to change the seat, so I decided to make an occasion of it. Without explaining why, I organized a special meal, put some wine on the table, placed some flowers in the centre and when the time came for the meal to be served I sat opposite my normal place. We are all creatures of habit, and this immediately threw the family into confusion as I had taken what was considered to be my youngest son's seat. I thought he would put a less of a fight than the others! I was right, he did not mind (too much) being asked to sit in 'my' seat. The first part of the meal was taken up with questions about the reason for the change. We all became so involved in discussing the ideas behind the move that time passed so quickly that I enjoyed an uninterrupted meal.

Since that time I have developed this idea in my approach for my own rehabilitation and have advocated to others the importance of thinking about every aspect of behaviour and breaking habits which have developed automatically over a period of time. Merely changing seats had not really got much to do with pain relief but it showed me that I had the power to try out small changes of behaviour and in return influence the way I felt. Moving seats, and the ensuing discussion, was a sufficient distraction from the discomfort which I would have expected.

Any small change that an individual makes has repercussions on the rest of those around them. It is like dropping a pebble into a pond and watching the ripples move outwards. Everybody is affected in some small way. Just as they have been adversely affected, perhaps unconsciously, by the changes when you retreated into your pain, any positive move from you will immediately be noticed. So, why not target a new change every day –

only a small one. It doesn't have to be earth-shattering. You might start by sleeping on the opposite side of the bed! Try it!

While working with a group of patients on this question of script change, Jean, aged 50, described a situation which made her very unhappy.

Jean had been suffering over five years from considerable pain in her back and legs and could not stand for long periods. Every evening she stood in the kitchen preparing the meal for herself and her husband aware all the time of the pain building up tension as she struggled on. When her husband came in from work and greeted her with a cheerful smile and a kiss the dam of tension burst and she found herself pushing him away snapping out: 'Can't you see I'm busy?'. The tone was set for the evening. He would quietly remove his coat, go into the sitting room and read his evening paper. Their meal would pass almost in silence. They would sit watching television hardly sharing a word until half way through the evening he would get up and go out to the pub leaving her in a state of tension and mixed feelings about her rejection of her husband's expression of affection but angry that she was left alone yet again.

Hearing all this reminded me of a time many years ago when I was 17, and working during the Christmas holiday period as a temporary postman. It was always dark by the time I finished my round in the village where I lived. Late one afternoon I had a parcel to deliver to a house at the far end of the village. As I stood in the darkened doorway trying to find the doorbell the door was flung open wide and a very naked lady threw her arms around me and kissed me. As she stuck to my cold, wet oilskins she realized I was not the real target and, embarrassed, untangled herself saying 'Oh, I'm, terribly sorry, I thought you were my husband – I wanted to give him a surprise!' In a state of shock I handed her the parcel and she disappeared indoors.

The story from my past was introduced to illustrate that there are all sorts of ways of greeting a returning spouse. The message contained in this story was simply 'Give him a surprise!' Jean got the message and the following week she turned up at the group full of excitement and with a rare sparkle in her eyes began to describe the results of her decision to make a change:

Instead of preparing the meal one evening, Jean spent the time doing her hair and her make-up, getting herself dressed up, complete with the earrings which her husband had bought her for Christmas. When she heard her husband's car she went outside to greet him. His response had been one of utter shock, first thinking that perhaps there had been some tragedy in the family and she was dressed up ready to go out to pay a sympathy visit. But then he saw that his wife was smiling! This was a sight he had not seen for many a long day!

Over a cup of tea, she told him she was trying to remove the barrier that had grown up between them. She could see that she was being unfair in letting her pain dictate the way she greeted him and realized how insensitive she had become about his feelings. Recognizing what was happening she wanted to clear the air. They chatted for some time discussing the unhappy changes that had taken place since the onset of her pain problem. Jean's husband was delighted to see his wife taking an interest in her appearance and actually enjoying the change. Since she had gone to all the trouble to dress up he thought they should go out to celebrate with a night out. This was the first evening they had been out together in a long time. Jean felt she had now broken through their barrier and the couple went on to devise a number of plans for making other changes in their lives. Over the specific question of meals, Jean and her husband realized that she was trying to keep up the practice of many years, when the children were at home and she was fit and strong, to have meals on the table when they returned from school or work. Now that they were on their own they could choose when to eat, and when they were ready could prepare the meal together and take their time to enjoy it. This suited them both as the husband had been feeling guilty knowing his wife was in pain and yet unable to find ways to offer a helping hand without making her feel inadequate.

Jean's efforts were admired by the group members and others began to share some of their experiences.

Tom who was 35, married, with a young family, had been out of work as a result of a back injury and pain which persisted for many months. After the children had gone to bed he and his wife had developed a pattern of sitting watching television, she knitting as she did so, alone on a settee, and he reclining in his armchair ostensibly watching the television but letting his mind drift. Usually these thoughts dwelt on his misfortune and how life had treated him so unfairly. It was almost although these negative thoughts were on an LP record, automatically switched on at various times of the day, making him more and more tense, more sorry for himself and feeling his pain more intensely to the accompaniment of the persistent clicking of his wife's knitting needles. They had reached a stage where they never talked to any purpose and his view of the future, for himself and for them both, was depressing. He opened up to the group as a result of listening to these stories about change and it seemed obvious to the others that what was needed was for him to take some action to get closer to his wife. 'Try sitting by her side on the settee tonight' was one suggestion. However, when he did this he was asked 'What the !! are you sitting there for?' This gave him the chance to explain what we had been discussing in the group and about breaking habits which were unhelpful. He described to his wife his feelings as he sat each evening in his own chair feeling isolated, brooding and becoming agitated as his tension and pain increased. He felt they were growing apart emotionally and the physical gap between their separate seats symbolized this. Tom explained how he felt excluded from his children. With good intentions, his wife frequently yelled at the children for 'bothering' him while he was in pain. He reminded his wife of the way things were before his illness and compared their present stagnant existence. They talked for three hours discussing their feelings about the situation they were both caught up in. They agreed that something must be done if they were to have a good future to look forward to. Together they began to develop ideas for making positive changes in their daily lives. Tom reported the whole incident back to the group who expressed their pleasure at his progress. Tom was particularly proud of a joint agreement between himself and his wife that he should ask his five-year old daughter to bring her new school reading book to him when she came home each day so that he could hear her read. This broke the pattern and enabled him to move on to doing more with the children including taking them swimming every Saturday morning. As well as improving his relationship with his children he benefited from the exercise.

Becoming aware of your present behaviour and the direction you wish to travel is often the first step towards identifying specific behavioural changes. Even though the changes you make may be small the results can be quite dramatic making an impact not only on the way you feel but setting off a chain of positive events for everyone associated with you.

Stepping over the obstacles to change

There can be obstacles in the way of your progress. These obstacles arise from negative, self-defeating thoughts and constant retreat into bad memories (just as Tom was doing). Just as you can set off a series of good events by making positive changes, so you can provoke a chain of negative behaviour persistently indulging in negative thoughts and attitudes. Remarks like 'I could never do that'; 'I can't'; 'I wouldn't dare'; 'I tried that once'; 'What's going to become of me?'; 'Will this pain never stop?' are common and trip off the tongue. When we are fit the limitations of negative thoughts may be minimal but when you have pain they can become dominant factors in determining whether or not you get better – or even try!

It is interesting that whenever I work on changing this aspect of the script and pose the question to patients: 'What was the most enjoyable thing you did last week?' an initial response, might be 'I had an enjoyable day out with the family . . . we drove to the seaside, had a picnic, had a long walk and it was great, but the day after I was creased with pain and couldn't get out of bed. It will be a long time before I do that again'. Notice that the word 'but' completely destroys the positive statement preceding it. Read the question again for yourself and observe that the question was simply 'What was the most enjoyable thing you did last week?' We are all guilty of using the word *but* to wipe out the benefit of any positive statements we might make. Just listen to yourself talking from time to time. Notice how often you use the word *but* and consciously ban it from your vocabulary. Get used to making simple, positive statements. It is sufficient to record occasions which were pleasurable and made you feel good. Unfortunately, people in chronic pain develop the habit of ignoring good things that happen to them and constantly focus on the bad things. People can often have six good days in every week, enjoying all sorts of activities in and around the home with family and friends, but one bad day can be enough to wipe from their memory all the good things that have happened.

It helps to keep a note of all the enjoyable things that happen to you and to remind yourself at the end of each day of the positive happenings. Talk about them, savour them and look forward to the next day. Good things can happen even on days when you have pain. Like today, for example. In terms of pain this has been a bad day – in terms of achievement this has been a very good day. As I complete this sentence I am aware that I have written well over 3000 words since this morning. I have enjoyed three good meals and in particular have had the chance to sample a new batch of strawberry jam freshly made by my wife. I have been for a two-hour walk along our local cliff path, enjoying some of the loveliest scenery in Britain, revelling in the sunshine and fresh air, spotting numerous varieties of sea birds and trying to identify the many wild flowers that grow in abundance on the cliffs. The ice cream on the way home just rounded off a very pleasant afternoon. Get used to recording the good things that happen and share them with as many people as possible and whilst you still have pain, it can be in the background and cease to dominate your life.

Do you remember Frank Spencer, the walking disaster from the television series *Some Mothers Do 'Ave 'Em*? He was well-known for his use of good, positive affirmations to give himself a boost and avoid being crushed by the pressure of life. He adopted for himself the well-known expression 'Every day and in every way, I am getting better and better'. The English language is full of such positive statements. Have fun finding them! There is one that goes 'Laugh and the world laughs with you, cry and you cry alone'. Let this be a warning!

Trouble is universal and everybody has their share – and they do not particularly want yours too so when you find yourself pouring out your troubles to someone who has asked how you are keeping, STOP! a moment. You are in danger of having that person avoid you in the future. Perhaps even worse, as you tell them your sorry tale your memory will find for you all the bad feelings that go along with it and these will stay with you, increasing your tension and increasing your pain. Similarly, if you are in the habit of brooding, slipping into bad memories, rehashing all the terrible things that have happened to you, and reliving bad experiences, you fire off all the negative emotions which use up valuable energy needed to aid your recovery. Get into the habit of becoming consciously aware of this tendency and switch your thinking to something positive and pleasant. In your imagination go to your special place, a place of warmth and comfort, which makes you feel good. Allow the positive memories to provoke positive feelings.

I frequently pull myself out of negative thinking and negative feelings by going in my imagination to a riverbank in mid-Wales and experience again all the sights and sounds and smells of that place, recalling the sight of the sand martins flying in and out of the river banks, seeing again the sunlight sparkling on the river in front of me, feeling the breeze ruffling my hair and being aware of the clouds scudding across the sky creating shadows on the mountains at the head of the valley. Everybody has a special place they can go to when necessary. Find yours, and go there frequently.

Anger

One of the most disabling emotions that anyone can have is anger. Just as your mind is often clouded by old thoughts, old fears and old expectations, leaving no room to think of the future, it can also harbour resentment and the tendency to find someone to blame for your misfortune. When you are feeling good difficulties you may have experienced with particular people may be shrugged off easily. When things are not going well it is possible to dwell irrationally on real or imagined slights suffered at their hands and blow them up out of all proportion and you can generate a high degree of emotion just by thinking about them. Strong emotions produce strong physical sensations increasing the pulse rate, increasing the blood pressure, causing more acid to be produced in the stomach, producing more tension – and again – producing more pain.

I have found that anger is a strong element in most pain sufferers I have worked with. It is often not recognized as anger, or the anger may even be denied by people with pain who have a great deal to be angry about. I was angry about the fact that my problem not only stopped progression in my career – but stopped it altogether. I was angry because . . . I lost the ability and the pleasure of playing football . . . or even watching it! I was angry because . . . I lost the ability to walk . . . to concentrate and enjoy reading and I was angry about the loss of so many things too numerous to mention, when I still had so much of my life ahead of me. However, I did not recognize my wretched feelings and inner discomfort as anger. So many people with pain do not recognize or express their anger straightforwardly. There is a tendency to displace it perhaps by exploding at an unsuspecting member of the family over something trivial, slamming doors as a way of protest. These things can happen when your anger is suppressed to bursting point. If you are suppressing anger you can be on edge, find yourself taking life too seriously, fighting tears, being unable to laugh at life's absurdities, indulging in long periods of silence, and if someone offends you, you can find yourself being inhibited in your ability to express legitimate anger directly at the person responsible and instead smoulder away, feeling resentment and hatred for the offender.

People with pain very rarely talk about their anger, may not even accept there is anger, and the unconscious attempts to suppress it are instrumental in creating a barrier between the person and those who may be in a position to offer help. Anger, just like anxiety and fear, is energy-consuming and disabling and it can turn inwards to eat away at your strength. It can ferment and grow, feeding your tension and discomfort. This is destructive and above all depresses the spirit and the will to change. It poses the biggest obstacle of all to getting rid of your pain.

It took me a long time to recognize this and I only got in touch with my anger with the help of Helen, a member of the Spiritual Healers' Association who worked regularly with the patients on the Pain Programme at Walton Hospital. She helped me to get in touch with the anger about all the things I have mentioned, to talk about them and to expel all the negative feelings that I had about the loss of my health. She was able to do this in such a way that the energy that I had been using to fuel my anger was released and directed towards my recovery. For example, at the end of a long session during which a great deal of negative feeling had been released, I felt a great surge of energy which I was able to direct towards walking for the first time in five years, without aid, from one side of the room to the other.

You may need help from someone skilled at releasing strong negative feelings and channelling them positively and this help is available to you from people trained in this area. In the meantime assess for yourself whether anger is at the root of some of your difficulties. It is easy to deny anger, saying you are not angry when in fact you are. Whether you deny it or not, *get in touch with the source of your internal discomfort.* Try writing down the phrase: 'I am angry because . . .' and make a list of all those things which contribute to your anger.

If you have got pain you have every reason to feel anger. Anger does not mean you are a bad person. You have no need to feel guilty about it so forgive yourself for being angry. Express it and state the reasons for your anger. There is no need to fear being destroyed by it if you recognize the feeling and the reasons for it and accept that you *must* act positively to make yourself feel better.

Sometimes when working with patients who appear withdrawn, depressed and generally flat, I find it helpful to provoke them to express their anger. This may be the first outburst of any kind of feeling they have had in a long time. This can be a very positive way of helping a person out of their depression. You can help yourself in a number of ways by making a list as I have suggested, or by telling people when they make you angry so that they might change or modify their behaviour.

I said earlier that strong emotions produce physical sensations. In my work as a psychotherapist, I often ask people to try the following exercise:

Close your eyes, and begin to focus on something in your life that makes you unhappy. As you do so, be aware of the feelings inside you. Perhaps a tightness in the stomach muscles or in the chest or throat. As you become aware of these things, begin your diaphragmatic breathing and each time you breathe out, mentally tell yourself that you are letting go of all the feelings of hatred, resentment and anger. Continue in this way until the discomfort inside you eases and you begin to feel the warmth of relaxation spread throughout your body.

You may need to do this each day for a week or two to feel the effects but it will make you feel better, calmer and result in a release of energy that you can use positively. Doing this will also inoculate you against harbouring new resentments and negative feelings.

Who's pulling your strings?

Throughout your life you may have developed ways of relating to others that present major obstacles to change. Your attitudes and emotional responses may hinder your efforts to change some aspects of your life which are causing you stress or aggravation. It may be that your emotional responses and behaviour are not entirely in your control and as a result you may feel some inner discomfort which adds to your tension and, consequently, your pain. So, now is the time to think about whether you are really in control of your life. Try to identify the source of this control: other people; hangovers from the past; your previous learning; or attitudes and beliefs passed on to you as a child. Any of these things can be a major source of distress and guilt.

I have prepared a list of statements which may or may not apply to you. If you find that most of them do, then it is time to make changes for your own benefit. You may legitimately be prevented by circumstances from making potentially beneficial changes in terms of your pain, but it is important to acknowledge which aspects of living are contributing to your distress.

- I believe there may be something basically wrong with *me* which is making me unhappy.
- I feel guilty when I am having my own way, even over something trivial.
- I don't like to 'rock the boat' even when something does not seem right.
- I feel guilty when I shirk a domestic duty – neglect to clean the house, leave washing-up overnight, do not have meals ready on time.
- I feel uneasy if my partner does not have a meal ready for me when I come home.
- I think I should be able to cope with any situation and that it is a sign of failure to ask for help.

91

- I believe I am not allowed to show anger. I feel angry about my situation but feel I cannot talk about it.
- I feel guilty over spending money on myself unless I have the approval of someone else, otherwise I make excuses for it.
- I still seek approval, not just the advice, of parents for major decisions in my life.
- My mother or father comes to mind whenever I 'disobey' a rule they taught me as a child and I expect to be punished.
- I believe that all rules should be followed because they are made by people whose judgement is better than mine.
- I accept invitations to do things with friends or family even when I would rather not and then resent them for aggravating my pain.
- I attend meetings, weddings, funerals, social functions out of a sense of duty rather than because I want to.
- If I am enjoying myself I expect discomfort to follow automatically, so I turn down opportunities to go out.
- I resist new experiences and have not done anything different for more than a month.
- I feel guilty and uneasy if I am away from home too long and I feel upset when something disrupts my daily routine.
- I feel that others do not believe that my pain is as bad as I make out and I find myself talking about it frequently to convince them.
- I tackle DIY jobs because I think it is expected of me even although I know I am not up to it.
- I truly feel that sacrificing myself for others makes me a better person, even though it means ignoring my own needs.
- I jump up immediately to answer the doorbell or telephone; I drop everything else to respond to an immediate demand.
- I am staying in a bad relationship because I wouldn't know where to turn if I was alone.

People who are dominated and controlled in the ways listed are not always aware of it, or, if they are, are afraid to make any changes lest they diminish themselves in the eyes of others. Continually trying to please others is a sign of diminished self-esteem as well as being physically, mentally and emotionally exhausting. Your pain may not be directly caused by this aspect of your personality and behaviour – but it will not be helped by it. Always responding without question to requests to help with heavy work in the garden, babysit till midnight, a weekly baking for church coffee mornings, must put a strain on anyone with pain attempting to pace themselves. The pain management message involves being engaged in purposeful activity and keeping busy, but if you are going to keep busy it must be in doing the things *you* enjoy, when *you* want to do them.

Working on your self-esteem

If you have chronic pain, you share with others who suffer from long-term illness or chronic disability the danger that you will lose your self-esteem and confidence. As you grieve your loss of physical capacity, ability to work, to earn money, provide for a family, to enjoy social activity, or you feel sexually unattractive, then it can be expected that the emotions I have talked about earlier in the chapter will surface from time to time.

With chronic illness, you seem to work hard at rebuilding your life but with each set-back or recurrence of a problem you are faced once again with the possibility of loss and are reminded of all those things you have lost since your illness started. Your grieving starts all over again – so too does your anger and rage – and, in some people, feelings that they are so worthless they might as well give up and not even try to do those things which they know can help them. Many people make a start at rebuilding their lives but because the negative feelings have not been dealt with and laid to rest, they can find themselves sabotaging their own efforts. It is no fault of theirs, but it is a sign that these people need professional help to grieve and 'lay their ghosts'.

There are people who can help you in the same way that I was helped by Helen. Talking about your feelings is important and will help to remove much of the confusion and negativity which can so easily dominate your mind. No one is exempt from these feelings of worthlessness. I have to keep reminding myself daily of the things that I have set my mind on achieving and that this negative stage will pass. Then I will have enough energy to 'pick myself up, brush myself down, and start all over again'!

If you recognize that these powerful emotions are an obstacle to your progress, then talk to your doctor about them. Your doctor can arrange for you to have psychological help through the NHS if he or she feels this is appropriate. Seeking refuge in tranquillizers in an effort to solve your problem will not help.

Self-esteem means the value we put on ourselves, but it also comes from the way other people respond to us. Families and friends need to be sensitive to ways of showing that they continue to value you as a person and recognize your contribution to the family. If you are gong to make the changes you have set your mind on, then you and your family will need to come to terms with your feelings of loss, your confusion and anger, and work towards rebuilding your self-confidence. The process may not be easy and will take time, but you can make a start and recognize that self-esteem needs to be worked on throughout life.

Try making a list of 10 positive statements about yourself. Many people with pain find this very difficult at first and need some prompting, so find someone who knows you pretty well and ask them to help you compile the list. Ask them to be honest and be honest with yourself. You have many good qualities and these need to be expressed and you need the opportunity to demonstrate them – starting *now*!

7

Stepping Out –
Alone or with a Partner

If you are alone and working on a programme to manage your pain you need to be equipped with a good self-starter and develop a firm resolve to carry through your plans. You will at least have the advantage of being free of over-protection. If your pain has made you virtually housebound you may have decided to make things easier for yourself and others by leaving the door on the latch during the day to allow easy access for neighbours or helpers. Doing this underlines your 'invalid' status, so try keeping your door locked and make the effort to get to the door to welcome your visitors.

Avoid falling into the trap of sleeping late every day. Set yourself a timetable which ensures that *you* take the initiative to seek out company and activities. Do not wait for people to phone you to ask how you are but instead ring your friends from time to time to ask after their welfare, or better still make firm dates to visit them. Begin now to make your plans for each day, each week, each month. The ability to plan ahead marks out the difference between a healthy person and an unhealthy person so if you have stopped planning, take this as a sign that you need to make changes.

The most difficult time for me when managing my own pain was when I was alone following the death of my first wife. Looking back on that period I am convinced that I was helped by all the skills I had learned for managing my pain. I was glad that I had developed the habits of *positive thought, exercise, relaxation, absorbing activities, a regular sleeping pattern, involvement with other people* and *planning ahead*. From time to time I found myself, as a result of loneliness grief and pain combined, slipping back into self-pity and depression and there were occasions when I would wake up at 1 or 2 o'clock in the morning still sitting in front of the television set which had long ceased to transmit. It is at these times when you are thrown back on to your own resources and you are faced with the challenge of submission or fighting on. Losing a partner is difficult enough without the added burden of the pain. I am sure that many of you reading this book will be facing the same problems which I faced and so far you may not have found the encouragement to do something about your situation. The encouragement for you to make the change must come from within. You have to decide for yourself that you are going to make the best of the rest of your life. Your experiences will have told you that life is short and that everyone has a responsibility to live it to the full. If there is something in your own life which is stopping you from doing this then face up to it. Remember! A decision to make one small change may be all that is needed.

There are a number of practical things, in addition to relaxation and exercise, that you can do to make yourself more comfortable. Try rubbing the heels of your hands together vigorously until the friction heats them up and then place the heels of your hands over your closed eyes and sit quietly breathing into your diaphragm. This can be very soothing. You can also place the heated heels of your hands on any painful areas of your body which are accessible. It may be that if you feel around your body you will find cold spots, perhaps, for instance, over your hips or on your thighs. The heat from your hands will encourage blood flow and induce comfort in these areas. You might find it will help ease tension in the back of the neck.

Frequently I close the gate to my pain by finding a 'rubbing post' – the edge of a door, or even a tree, where I can gently ease away any discomfort in my back and shoulders.

Getting out and about

If you are able to get out of the house, do it with some purpose. Plan to go to places where you can meet people, perhaps a concert or an evening or day class run by your local authority. This is particularly important if you are able to sit for an hour quite comfortably. For those of you who can tolerate longer periods of sitting or travelling why not try one of your local coach companies who provide short breaks to somewhere interesting without the trouble of driving. These are often associated with hobbies, special events or shopping so you get the benefit of a change of scenery and faces with the added attraction of doing something different. If you have any particular interests you are likely to find them catered for in the

Residential Colleges which are run either privately or by local authorities throughout the country. They come under the auspices of the National Institute for Adult Continuing Education (NIACE) and provide day, weekend or weeklong courses with or without accommodation. Some of these require no previous knowledge of the subject and take into account disability problems. From my own experience, as both a student and tutor at these colleges, the atmosphere is friendly and relaxed, and the accommodation and food are of a high standard, and what is more the prices are low when compared with packages you can find at your local travel agents. (The usual package holidays can underline your single status, particularly in the evenings and in some of their organized activities.) I enjoyed the involvement with other people with similar interests so much that I found I was able to afford to plan to go on a course once a month. This was a real treat and did much to further my rehabilitation. It was on such a course that I met my present wife, but I am not suggesting this as a reason for going on these courses! The point I am making is that you must plan to get involved as much as possible with people, that you should pursue your own interests, and as you do, you will find that your problems cease to dominate your life.

You will have seen from the previous chapter just how concerned people with pain can be about the deterioration in relationships between themselves and their loved ones. It seems appropriate to pick up and consider in a positive way some of these issues so that you and your partner can begin to look constructively at practical measures for strengthening your relationship.

Even the strongest partnership can be tested thoroughly when one of the pair has a pain problem. It could be that rather than your problem being shared and halved it might multiply because your partner's resources and abilities to cope are stretched to the limit. The fit partner is often left feeling powerless to provide any comfort and perhaps be made to feel guilty about enjoying good health. This can often lead to an over-protective attitude involving fetching and carrying and taking on the household tasks. For example, breakfast in bed! No doubt it helps the sick one to remain comfortable for long periods. However, this kind of behaviour reinforces the 'sick' role and imposes even stricter limitations on the amount of activity the pain sufferer is involved in. In the end, the cossetting can hasten the immobility and consequent disability.

The problem then is how the partner can help without smothering. The following suggestions are meant to be taken as part of the general approach outlined in the rest of this book.

If both can accept the necessity for the pain sufferer to be reactivated, become more independent, and to develop a positive approach to life, then these suggestions should be helpful. The partner can become aware of the deep, often disabling feelings which the pain sufferer is reluctant to talk about and help them to acknowledge, talk about and grieve for the loss of their former life, job, sports, social activities, fitness. The two can work together in devising and planning ways to establish and meet targets. In particular, it is helpful to have a second opinion when you are planning to take up some activity which you have not done for some time because of your pain. It is all too easy to bite off more than you can chew in your enthusiasm to get going! Your partner can help to set realistic goals.

The partner's positive attitude for the future can be communicated in what is said – and the manner in which it is expressed. This positive action sets a good example. If you feel that communication in your family may be a stumbling-block, why not sit down together and examine any negative attitudes and statements which are limiting progress?

Earlier I have referred to the adverse effects on all members of the family when one of them is dominated by illness. The sick partner in particular may have retreated from decision-making, disciplining the children and for a long time been on the receiving end of various aspects of care, and it may be that the healthy partner has found opportunities for an independent social life as a release from the extra responsibility. Everyone around assumes you have abdicated all responsibility and it might come as a shock when part of your rehabilitation involves taking back the reins.

It is possible that patterns have been set which are then difficult to alter. If problems have gone on for a number of years the recovering partner may find, if they expect to resume the relationship from where it left off, that the partner's outlook has changed and they can still feel very much left behind. For example Peter, as he was getting better, set as his target a visit to the Social Club he and his wife had frequented together for twenty years before the onset of his pain problem three years earlier. He had not even considered the possibility that his wife might not want to go back to that particular place and was devastated when she said in no uncertain terms that she would not set foot there again just to sit with a group of women for the whole evening while their men lounged around drinking ale at the bar! She insisted Peter took her out to a restaurant. Peter was forced to consider that he was going to have to make bigger changes than he thought. It is the realization that the world has moved on while you have stayed still that can be very difficult to cope with.

This realization, rather than making you feel upset or guilty, can in fact help you to look a lot further ahead in your recovery and make you take stock of every aspect of your life, and this includes, perhaps for the first time in a long time, taking a real interest in your partner's wellbeing. It may force you to respect the way in which your partner has adjusted to difficult circumstances and has continued to live a positive life. Each of you will need to consider providing space for the other to participate in activities together or separately. One way your partner can help in the early stages is to encourage you to get inolved in an active social life, in hobbies, pastimes and outings, taking reasonable care to see that the activities are manageable. There is no reason why couples should not participate in the residential and day courses referred to earlier. You and your partner may go together, share accommodation and mealtimes but choose different subjects. Such activities can help extend horizons for both of you and provide new topics of interest in conversation thus making it easier to communicate on a level other than that relating to pain and suffering.

Good communication between partners can be enhanced in a number of ways and this can apply equally well to couples where illness is not the problem. These suggestions can help to establish more physical comfort for the pain sufferer and revive the sense of partnership.

Massage

Although you may benefit from professional therapeutic massage from time to time, this is not absolutely necessary. Investment in a small bottle of scented oil or massage lotion will enable your partner to administer gentle massage to any part of the body where you find it comforting (warm hand, and oil first!). This will be much more beneficial than having breakfast in bed as it will have a direct influence on your pain and enjoyment. Your partner will be delighted to have been instrumental in improving your feelings of comfort even for only a short time. Remember the gate theory of pain and how rubbing or stroking can close the gate to the pain messages. This is what is happening. Working together in this way may help to break down or prevent possible barriers being set up between you.

Sometimes you may feel that there are parts of your body which are too sore to massage. Your partner can still help, particularly when trying to get off to sleep which can be a difficult time, by placing the palm of his or her hand gently on your sore spot. It helps if your partner has learned diaphragmatic breathing in order to develop a slow, relaxed breathing rhythm. This will help to induce relaxation in both of you and you will find that you can draw comfort from the combination of warm hand and steady breathing.

Also, breathing in this way, your pain can be eased if your partner holds your wrist near the area of the pulse, and places the other hand in the nape of your neck. This serves to reduce tension and relieve pain. This is also an exercise which the pain sufferer can do for his or her fit partner at those times when perhaps he or she has become over-tired or has a headache. It is a very good thing for the partner with pain to reciprocate if only to demonstrate to the fit partner just how comforting this can be, and by doing so the pain sufferer will also feel the calming, soothing effects.

There are many areas of the body which can be stimulated to bring about pain relief. Gentle massage of the temples and the nape of the neck on either side of the spine is useful in the relief of head or face pain. Aching shoulders can be eased by gentle massage at shoulder level about two inches on either side of the spine. Similarly, the back can be massaged with the fingers along its whole length by exerting gentle pressure either side of the spine. This is particularly effective right at the base of the spine where it is possible to induce deep relaxation and even a sleepy feeling. Many people enjoy massage of the feet but if you are like me, your feet may be over-sensitive. It helps if firm massage is used in this case so that it doesn't tickle.

So establish this two-way contact through gentle stroking, massage, or just laying on of hands and recognize the contribution each is making to the other. And remember, it is often better to give than to receive so don't let it be all one-way! You may even find it fun!

Lovemaking and allowing yourself to be touched

Frequently even a happy, close relationship is disturbed either because of pain or because of fear of damage and therefore more pain. Similarly, the fit partner may not wish to appear inconsiderate and may seek protection from possible rejection by inhibiting sexual overtures. It is understandable that the pain sufferer whose energies are taken up in coping with the pain will, from time to time, be unresponsive and even rejecting. Therefore it may be easier to develop an over-protective attitude and to deny normal sexual needs. Be reassured that having sexual intercourse will not in itself damage you. However, it is to be expected that you may find it difficult to relax weak, tense and painful muscles sufficiently and this is where the suggestions in earlier paragraphs can be particularly helpful. Like all activity you need to build up the strength and stamina. You can start by having earlier nights and allow time for a warm bath and a period of deep relaxation to warm your body thoroughly. A number of patients I worked with had problems over being touched and this can be very off-putting to a partner. Pain often brings with it a high degree of sensitivity to being touched, and light, stroking movements which had previously been pleasurable, can now produce acute discomfort. Not all touch is unpleasurable even in those over-sensitive areas and it may be that stronger, firmer pressure over a larger area can overcome this localized discomfort. Have you perhaps developed the habit of 'guarding' yourself so much that you guard yourself against pleasure as well as pain?

You may not be so athletic as you once were but there are other ways to show your partner that you enjoy the closeness of lovemaking. Perhaps all that is required is a change to a side-by-side position which is less tiring. You enjoyed experimenting in the beginning so there is no reason why you should not enjoy the re-learning.

8

Practical Ways to Get Going

Originally I planned to call this chapter 'Use it or Lose it' but rejected the title as my aim is to encourage rather than to frighten. Nevertheless, the statement is true and the pain sufferer has to face this fact. *Prolonged inactivity produces disability.*

A common characteristic of people with pain is that they have restricted their social life. Some no longer go shopping, driving, playing sports, walking, going to the theatre, eating out, playing with the children, travelling on trains, buses or planes. If this has happened already or you are aware that it is happening, then it is important that you personally take the trouble to work out how pain has affected your life and your activities.

This chapter will focus on practical suggestions for coping with some of the activities just mentioned using the principles of Relaxation, Planning, Goal-setting and Targeting. You really have to ask yourself: 'How is this pain affecting my life?' and also: 'What have I stopped doing because of my pain?'

I am assuming that anyone who is locked into pain has a deep desire to do as much as possible to escape, provided someone can show the way. It is important to accept the philosophy that if pain is inevitable, it is better to have it as a result of doing something rather than doing nothing. This chapter sets out the route. The aim is to progressively give the brain so much work to do that pain ceases to be its sole preoccupation and becomes just one of many tasks it has to perform. Experience shows that once a person starts on the journey there is a progressive reduction in pain.

If you are locked into chronic pain then it is likely you will be spending a great deal of time reclining or lying down. But the longer we spend in this position the more likely it is that muscles will lose tone and become wasted. What's more, the pain, which originated in one part of the body, becomes generalized giving feelings of bruising, stiffness and acute discomfort through the whole body. Therefore, when returning to any activity after a long interval, there is a need for progressive re-training. Muscles need to be prepared and the person in pain needs to be helped to cope with the fear and anxiety surrounding the move from recumbent immobility to full mobility.

In order to begin to cope with this problem – and assuming that you want to become mobile – let us start with the notion of self-monitoring.

Monitoring yourself

You should begin by recording information about the amount of time you spend lying down, reclining, sitting, walking, washing, eating, preparing and cooking meals, shopping, reading, watching TV, meeting friends, playing with children or any other activities engaged in during the day. Ideally, a two-day-per-page diary is most suited to this task. If it helps, make a note of how you spend each hour!

Your diary is going to be very useful. It is going to show you just how much progress you make day by day. I suggest that you select an activity that you have neglected for some time and, each day, record what you are doing to re-establish this aspect of your life. Quite simply, set yourself a target and aim to reach it – slowly but surely, one step at a time.

The strategies outlined assume that at the moment you are not very active so the targets are set at a low level. Some of you may be fitter than others so you can start at a level which you think is comfortable for you. We are all individuals each having a different problem and will progress at different rates. Sitting and walking are basic to most activities, so we will start with these.

Sitting

It would seem to be a contradiction in terms to describe sitting as an 'activity'. However, as explained earlier, if you have been accustomed to be in a reclining or lying position, your muscles will have been weakened. It seems an even greater contradiction to start by demonstrating how to learn to sit still! But this is where we are going to start.

Find a chair, preferably one that you have never sat in before as it is important to choose a chair in which you have not previously experienced failure or discomfort. As in the illustration in the section on Posture (see p. 51), it should support you completely from the top of your head, through your back, your buttocks and your thighs. If necessary prop yourself with pillows behind and around you. Sit with your bottom well back, with your spine straight, your feet firmly planted on the floor and your hands resting lightly on your thighs. This is a balanced sitting position.

Start by practising your breathing into the diaphragm. Slow down your breathing and now decide how long you are going to sit on this first occasion. If your diary shows that you have actually been accustomed to sitting, rather than reclining, for no more than 5 minutes at a time, then aim to sit for 5 minutes only, irrespective of whether you feel comfort or discomfort. This is important for your recovery. Any discomfort you feel is only related to your muscles being in an unaccustomed position. You are not doing yourself any harm or further injury. While you are sitting there breathing you might include another useful activity. For example, you can add to the adventure by closing your eyes, continuing to practise your diaphragmatic breathing and clearly fix in your mind some pleasurable activity that you can enjoy at the end of a week of progress.

Think of what you could do one week from this moment if you have progressively increased the amount of time you sit each day.

Progress in sitting comfortably can be rapid and I suggest you have several periods of sitting in this way, each day, increasing the amount of time you sit on each occasion. For example in the first hour sit for 5 minutes. In the second hour, 10 minutes, in the third hour, 20 minutes. Use a relaxation tape to help you extend your sitting time. You will be pleasantly surprised at how quickly your ability to sit comfortably returns. My experience has taught me that people who have lost the ability to sit, find that by the end of the first week they can sit, with interludes for exercise, meals and other breaks, from 9 o'clock in the morning until 5 o'clock in the evening. Very frequently, using hypnosis, I have helped patients to sit comfortably for two hours where previously their sitting time had been a matter of minutes. So, while you are sitting there thinking about what you can do in a week's time, make a firm resolve to do something at the end of that week that you have not done in a long long time. Perhaps you could arrange to go to the pub or to visit a neighbour for a cup of tea. Decide in advance how long you will stay, tell your friends that you will leave at the time arranged and that you will stay longer next time. Do *not* make the mistake which is frequently made, of staying longer because you are comfortable and then finding you become overwhelmed by discomfort and feel a failure as a result.

Don't forget, relaxation and diaphragmatic breathing is the key to sitting comfortably. These points can be easily forgotten once you get involved with others in company. Rehearse all this in your imagination, in particular, imagine the feeling of completing the task successfully. Experience in your imagination the pleasure and pride of success. Immediately you have practised and succeeded in your imagination, make arrangements to carry out your intention in reality and continue to equip yourself with daily practice.

Your first adventure over, start planning your next! Begin to plan other more demanding activities. Always set yourself a realistic time limit for social occasions. You can plan to go out for a meal knowing that a meal usually takes about an hour and a half, so make it a target. Treat yourself to a meal in a restaurant. Make it an occasion!

Remember, even though you may feel pain when you get home, you would have had it anyway if you had stayed in, so don't be tempted to make it an excuse not to do it again!

Five months after I had been lying down for most of the day and I was on the road to recovery I set myself the target of travelling by train to London from North Wales once every two weeks to sit for a weekend studying and listening to lectures on psychotherapy for up to eight hours a day on the Saturday and Sunday. I found that I survived the rail journey by using a Walkman, loading in a relaxation tape when I got on the train, listening to that and going into deep relaxation while it was on. I would then walk down the train to the buffet car and spend half an hour taking refreshment and then back to the Walkman for relaxing music or a hypnosis tape. I did this journey regularly over a period of two years, all the while getting progressively more mobile and more comfortable.

It is important to get to grips at an early stage with extending your comfort whilst sitting, as many people with pain are put off from enjoying a rich social life and holidays because of their fears of discomfort. As you get better, plan trips to the theatre or to concerts or to the club or other places of entertainment. Always remember to plan for success! If you do have a set-back don't treat it as a disaster – just a hiccup. After all, when you were a baby learning to walk you fell over many, many times. You picked yourself up and started all over again.

Walking

Walking is central to most other activities. I have already indicated just how good walking is for strengthening leg muscles, back muscles, helping with circulation and general body functioning. Confidence in walking opens the doors to most of our social and essential daily tasks. No one expects that a person who has spent a long time sitting or lying down in the pain state will initially have muscles which are strong enough for walking long distances so progressive physical exercise is basic to establishing general fitness for walking. In my experience, many people with chronic pain develop a fear or deep anxiety about walking and it helps to have someone to encourage you at all times. When you first start walking it is possible that you will experience pain after a short time but remember, pain does not necessarily equate with doing yourself an injury.

When I was first getting going I would turn right outside my gate, walk 50 or 60 yards along the road and find that I was overcome with pain, tiredness and weakness, and I took this as a signal to stop. I would rest awhile and return home utterly discouraged by my failure to make progress. It doesn't take many experiences like this to condition a person to expect the onset of pain at a particular point in a walk. If this has been your experience then think about getting a friend to take you somewhere new. Plan to go to a local beauty spot or somewhere interesting where you have never walked before, or perhaps a place where you have been before when you were well and where your friend has never been. It will add interest to the trip if you are thinking about showing your friend some of the things that you enjoy about the place. The important point is that you go to a place which does not remind you of failure – the more beautiful and interesting the better.

On the first occasion plan to walk for no more than 5 minutes (or more if your functioning is better than the low level of mobility I have assumed). If you feel any discomfort at all, remember your breathing exercises. The aim on this first occasion is to be successful by setting a time-limit. Give yourself every opportunity to succeed. Success breeds success.

On the next occasion extend the time limit, knowing that you can do 5 minutes comfortably, but here again, be careful not to take too big a bite all at once, perhaps 8–10 minutes is sufficient on this occasion. Concentrate on the fact that you are out to enjoy yourself, to enjoy the scenery, to enjoy the sights and sounds and to enjoy the feeling of the fresh air on your face. Again, remember the breathing and relaxation. Relaxation before and after the walk will help to reduce any anxiety or pain.

Initially, choose reasonably flat, even ground to walk on and if you have feet which are sensitive, as many pain patients do, make sure you have footwear that has thick cushion soles; preferably also wear a good pair of walking socks. Wear light, warm clothing. It is better to have layers of light material rather than one heavy layer. Heavy clothing can present problems to people with back, neck and leg pains in particular. In recent years I have discarded a heavy sheepskin coat, a tweed overcoat and a duffle coat. In their place I have substituted lightweight padded clothing.

After several successful excursions, gradually increase your time limits and at the same time be more adventurous in terms of walking further, even though you may feel discomfort. When you are walking comfortably for 20 minutes remind yourself that you are probably walking as much or perhaps even further than the average pain-free individual who travels to work in a car, sits in an office all day and comes home to spend an evening slouched in front of the television, so be proud of yourself! Don't forget that you can reward yourself during a walk in many different ways – perhaps calling in for a drink, alcoholic or otherwise, en route. Try varying your pace. As you become more proficient try increasing your pace for about fifty yards or so, lengthening your stride. Always remember your breathing exercises and develop the knack of breathing into your diaphragm all of the time. It is unfortunate that so many people, as they get older, get into the practice of ambling along. This is possibly because they are in no hurry. It is a habit to be avoided! A brisk walk for half an hour each day will do you much more good than strolling aimlessly along for the same length of time.

I had always been a keen walker so losing my mobility was a great disappointment which I felt even more because I sensed I was also denying my family a great deal of pleasure. We had always walked together locally in North- and mid-Wales, and in the Lake District. As I grew more confident with my developing walking skills, as well as driving, which I shall come to shortly, I decided to reward myself with a weekend trip to the Lakes, a reasonable two-hour drive from my North Wales home. Imagine what a great achievement it was to actually walk around Grasmere Lake, a distance of approximately four miles! Most of it is flat, easy walking apart from one short section. It took from ten o'clock in the morning to four in the afternoon and included stops for drinks, a picnic, admiring the scenery and taking photographs, a relaxation session and chats to fellow walkers we met on the way. At this time I was behaving as any other walker might and at the end of the day I was able to take stock and compare myself with the person who months before had spent most of every day confined to the house and this gave me a real sense of achievement and marked the release from my imprisonment.

So far, I have talked about walking on flat, even ground and now it is time to apply the same principles to gradients and uneven ground. If you will forgive me using myself as an example again, I decided to tackle our local mountain, Moel Fammau, all 2000 feet of it! It took 18 months to reach the top! This meant visiting the mountain once every few weeks and walking five minutes to begin with and being content with the distance covered in that time. Remember it is often more difficult to come down a mountain than it is to go up. There is an unaccustomed strain put on leg and foot muscles which have not been used for some time. On each occasion I increased the time by a few minutes, until – eighteen months later, and with much joy – I reached the top of the mountain which I had first climbed when I was six years old! Of all the times I had climbed it, this was the best. This was New Years' Day 1987.

Walking for pleasure is now an essential part of my daily activity. By the Spring of 1989 I was able to join a group of fit people walking 12 miles a day in the French Alps.

Walking stimulates the release of endorphins, maintains general fitness, brings spiritual uplift and increasing confidence. In fact, I think it is so important that I organized some groups of patients at various stages of recovery to undertake walks in the country. We applied the principles I have outlined and these were reinforced by the support of the group. In some cases such an activity was the first social occasion they had enjoyed for a long time.

Walking can still be a problem for many in places like super-markets, shopping malls, libraries, art galleries – in fact anywhere where it is not possible to maintain a steady rhythmic pace. The slow progress through shops, particularly when crowded, takes its toll and you may only be able to do this type of walking for limited periods. However, it is worth persevering. I will return to this in the section on shopping.

Driving

The same principles apply in getting back to driving. Assuming that you are starting off at a very low level of tolerance, you could follow this plan which is based on the one recommended to patients on the Pain Management Programme at Walton Hospital.

Step 1: Sit in the car and get used to it. All you have to do on this occasion is get yourself comfortably seated. Go through a relaxation exercise while sitting in the driver's seat. Remember, if you have not driven for some time, then you are losing nothing by taking time over your rehabilitation.

Step 2: Sit in the car and turn on the engine. Remember that it is essential to have the garage doors open if you are sitting in a stationary car with the engine on. On this occasion, if you have a driveway, just get used to the controls again, driving forward and reversing. Take note of the manoeuvres you can do comfortably.

Step 3: Drive around the block with a friend.

Step 4: Drive around the block alone.

Step 5: Drive around a well-known area for 10 minutes.

Step 6: Drive around a well-known area for 15 minutes.

Step 7: Drive around a well-known area for 20 minutes.

Step 8: Take a drive into the countryside.

Step 9: Take a drive around town on a quiet day.

Step 10: If it applies, take a drive to the town centre.

Spread these steps over several days. Essentially try to make the task easy at first, then increase the difficulty gradually, in small steps. It is important that you succeed and feel the pleasure of succeeding at each step. You may find that your pain level rises at times but persevere and confront your pain. Remember your relaxation skills and use them, the pain will not feel so bad. You are not going to do yourself any damage. Tell yourself that, with relaxation, in time the pain will pass off.

I find it is useful when I have to stop for any reason, say for traffic lights, to check my sitting position and my breathing. If my breathing is high in the chest I relax by breathing into the diaphragm. Diaphragmatic breathing *always* releases tension and reduces pain.

As your driving progresses it is wise not to be foolhardy and drive over a long journey in one big effort. Wherever you go you need to be able to arrive feeling reasonably fresh and able to enjoy the focus of your journey, whether it is work, or pleasure. Make a habit of not driving for more than an hour at a stretch before taking a break, relaxing fully, getting out and stretching your legs. If you have a partner who drives, then longer journeys can be broken up between you with each of you taking an hour at the wheel. This really does extend your driving distance at the same time as extending your horizons and enabling you to relax as a passenger. This is an area where you must allow your partner to share the work and where you must learn to relax while she or he is doing it.

Housework

Housework is an essential part of everyday life – for men as well as women – and what I have to say applies equally to both. A man who has pain and is at home all day while his partner is working can make housework a useful and rewarding part of his rehabilitation as well as easing the burden on his partner. This can mean a role reversal in the home with the man taking on the household chores and shopping, as it was in my own case. Psychologically, many women measure their worth by the way they manage their household, the quality of the meals, the brightness of the rooms, the dust-free carpets and furniture, gleaming worktops, etc. However, patients generally complain that they have difficulty with bed-making, vacuuming, ironing, and standing in the kitchen. Again, the principle is to take each task and break it down into small manageable parts.

Getting back to housework means sitting down, preferably with your partner, and working out a plan for sharing household duties during the initial training period at least. Plan to take one task at a time, for example, vacuuming, and do one room only. Then do some relaxation exercises and, having had a break, take another task, for example, peeling potatoes. When this task is complete divert yourself by taking a walk round the garden or doing some physical exercise and then come back and perhaps prepare other vegetables. Gradually build up the amount of work you do each day. If you have been used to vacuuming the house from top to bottom at a particular time each week, then make it a regular practice to do only one room on any one day. If you have been used to cleaning windows all around the house, get used to doing only one at a time.

Discussions with patients at the hospital are often most lively on the subject of housework and I find that women in particular, resist these ideas vigorously, being ruled very much by their own idea of what they *ought* to be doing. There is a tendency for the houseproud person to struggle to keep the high standard they set themselves. Remember, *ought* and *should* are part of the negative thinking process that we have already discussed. It is essential to take a much more relaxed attitude to housework and to discuss with family members how they might make a contribution. Remember that no one finds it pleasant to live with someone who has used up all their energy on household tasks, gets locked into pain, and becomes irritable and poor company.

A good example of this was Gwen:

One day, during a discussion at the hospital, Gwen looked out of the window and suddenly became very tense. Her face twisted in horror. She was watching the hospital window cleaner. I asked her why she had suddenly become so tense and she blurted out: 'But he's not doing the bloody corners! – you can't do windows and leave the bloody corners!' This became the focus of our discussion and it appeared that Gwen was not only a very conscientious housewife – but a martyr! constantly tidying up after her family, vacuuming any crumbs after a meal, cleaning and polishing all day long, plumping cushions. Anyone who left a newspaper on a chair would provoke criticism from her. She constantly nagged her family, complaining that they were inconsiderate and . . . if they only knew how much pain she had to suffer then they would do a lot more to help her, etc. However, she constantly rejected any ideas they put forward about making a positive contribution so gradually they left her to her suffering and just ignored all her complaints.

Following our discussion she agreed that over a weekend she would ask each family member in turn to assist with one task around the house. It took a lot of encouragement to get her to do this but on her return the following Monday she was pleased because she found that as a result of making these requests there had been a much more relaxed atmosphere in the house. She had made more time for relaxation and her husband had noticed that for the first time for a couple of years her face had actually relaxed into a smile.

Another patient, where housework figured prominently in her problem, was Judith, 70 years old:

Judith had had moderate pain for a few years but it had not stopped her looking after her home and family and leading a full social life. Her real problem started when her husband retired and gradually took over many of 'her' jobs: shopping, window cleaning, vacuuming. He was determined to keep himself busy during his retirement. With good intentions he insisted that, to save her any discomfort, he would make himself as useful as possible. Gradually Judith became more and more immobile and incapable of doing the jobs that she had done so well during forty years of marriage. It took time for both partners to accept that the husband had in fact made his wife redundant and that her rehabilitation depended on him being less protective. They needed help to establish a new partnership for their joint retirement.

Shopping

In discussion with many patients I find shopping is not seen as a problem. Men with pain opt out of shopping and so do many women who have a partner to pick up the groceries. But this will just not do! Like housework, shopping is an essential part of daily living and is not to be left for somebody else to do.

It is very rarely that shops offer a personal delivery service and in most supermarkets seats may only be provided at the exit for customers awaiting taxi collection. Although special arrangements are made to assist the non-ambulant, wheelchair customers, there are many more chronic pain sufferers, perhaps not recognized as such, who are attempting to maintain normal living by doing their own shopping and who would benefit tremendously from just having one or two seats at intervals round the store. This would allow them to recharge their energy and therefore extend their tolerance of shopping. Modern supermarkets cover a vast area and they can be forbidding places to the person with chronic pain. Personally, I find that this is the most demanding of all shopping.

Breaking down the task of shopping into small parts is important:

Visit 1: Go to one bay only, up one side and down the other then straight to the quietest checkout. If you are kept waiting, then use some of the relaxation techniques discussed earlier, breathing or visualization.

Visit 2: Do two bays. Leave by the quietest checkout and remember breathing and relaxation.

Gradually increase the amount of time spent in the supermarket and remember that you can ask for assistance with packing and for carrying things out to your car. This is part of the normal service in most supermarkets now. They cannot help you if they do not know you need help!

An alternative approach is to choose one section of the supermarket on the first visit, say the cheese section or the vegetable section or frozen foods, and gradually increase the number of sections you visit on any one occasion. Remember that the principle is to break down the task into small parts and gradually increase the difficulty of the task.

For other types of shopping, say for clothes or shoes, decide in advance how much time you are going to spend. Initially choose half an hour and decide what you are going to focus on and which store you are going to. Do some research to find out whereabouts in the

113

store you are likely to find what you are looking for and avoid shuffling round in the crowds being jostled until you chance to find what you are after. Gradually extend the amount of time you allow yourself for shopping but always follow the principle of planning your trip to include a break for coffee or lunch and relaxation. At Christmas-time I find it helpful to take my custom away from the city centres into small country towns where I can combine a day of walking with shopping. This takes a lot of hassle out of the task and in fact adds to the enjoyment of Christmas especially as small towns in summer holiday areas offer many bargains at this time. Craft fairs are another good, civilized way to shop for gifts and are often sited in pleasant villages.

Looking after children

Coping with children is demanding at the best of times. Many patients with pain are upset that their ability to cope with their own children or their grandchildren, or other young members of their family has been eroded. They recognize their fears that they may be hurt if they get involved physically in any way. They recognize their impatience and irritability and see that they have withdrawn from many situations where children are involved. There are some people who are in unfortunate situations which are made worse by their pain.

Maureen, aged 28, was a single-parent with two children aged 4 and 6. She had a chronic pain condition of the neck and shoulder which was aggravated by the necessary physical involvement with her young children. Her distress made her irritable and intolerant of their normal activities. She had not lost any real mobility because her task kept her so active and there was no one else to help her look after the children. Maureen was helped by learning to relax and to extend her range of social activity, in particular, she was helped to join in with a group of other young mothers and children so that the whole family could spend a relaxed few hours together. With encouragement she involved herself and the children in other community activities such as swimming and outings. She found that the tensions built up within her and the family through being confined to home were more easily coped with on neutral ground.

Many parents find this task of re-establishing normal relationships with their children quite daunting, especially if they have 'dropped out' of the caring, disciplining, or companionship role. With recovery it is important to sit down and plan and target aspects of behaviour towards children that you would like to develop on the way to getting back to the normal parenting relationship. You could decide to get involved in just a small way at first – reading a bedtime story, going on a trip, or planning an activity together. In my own case, I actually found a number of advantages from being in the chronic pain state in relation to my children. As I was at home all day I was considered by them to be available for advice and guidance on homework and study at any time. During school holidays I had their company and we were able to do many things together which I would have missed out on if I had been engaged in my usual frenzied activities as a working father. Also, when I was with them I was not so conscious of my pain.

If you can get physically involved, even in a limited way, with children, it can stop you from losing your mobility and the children will see you in quite a different light and value your companionship even more.

Do it yourself

Many people who do home decorating seem to follow a pattern of clearing out a room, preparing surfaces and getting on with painting or papering. They will often start the process early one morning over a Bank Holiday carrying on until they finish in the early hours or until they drop – whichever is first! This is not to be recommended for the recovering chronic pain patient! Do-it-yourself, like all the other activities we have talked about, needs to be planned and targets set with the idea of completing the task successfully by taking a number of small manageable steps. It may mean that rooms are upset just slightly longer and the family may have to tolerate domestic disruption for a few days rather than a few hours.

Just imagine, if you have been fretting for months or even years at your inability even to think about tackling decorating a room, what an achievement it can be to complete a decorating task.

Harry was concerned that he had lost his masculinity because he had to sit fretting whilst his wife donned the overalls, did the painting and the papering. Some people might be delighted at the prospect but not so Harry. Together we devised a plan:

1. Harry asked for assistance from the family in clearing the hall of the small pieces of furniture. The hall was chosen as the first target because it was mainly free from furniture and was small enough to tackle with confidence.

2. Harry and his son washed the walls and paintwork.

3. Harry organized the materials needed to do the job.

4. The family went out and Harry sat down with a relaxation tape and relaxed completely for half an hour.

5. He began to apply a coat of emulsion paint to the walls. He worked for 10 minutes, checked out how he was feeling, and had a change of activity. He walked around the garden for 5 minutes.

6. Harry returned to painting for 20 minutes.

7. He made himself a cup of coffee, sat down and practised diaphragmatic breathing for 10 minutes.

8. Another 20 minutes of painting.

9. Approximately 2 hours had elapsed since the family left home and Harry could assess just how much work he had done. Normally the emulsion painting job would have been completed in this time but surveying his work Harry could see that already he had completed more than half his task and that all he needed were three more spells of approximately 20 minutes to finish. He was feeling reasonably fresh but ready for a lunch break and another period of 30 minutes complete relaxation.

10. Harry resumed, doing three periods of 20 minutes with an interval of 10 minutes between each, making another 1½ hours. That was his work schedule for that day. It had been completed comfortably with the aim of producing maximum satisfaction for Harry and leaving him enough energy to enjoy the rest of the day to celebrate his achievement. I would like to be able to say that

Harry cleared up as he went and did not leave his brushes in the kitchen sink!

He repeated his schedule on the following day when he tackled the woodwork. (Purists would have done it the other way round!)

This approach has helped Harry and many others to tackle successfully a whole range of do-it-yourself activities. Following the principles of breaking down the tasks into small parts and setting time limits it is possible to achieve far more than many fit people. I have been helped considerably since I bought an electric screw-driver and an electric jigsaw. These have taken the strain off my muscles and helped me to continue to work for longer periods, and without pain.

9

Keeping Going at Work

Like many other people you may be attempting to carry on at work whilst coping with pain and with the burdens of fear and anxiety that go with it. You may be worried about admitting weakness and at the same time afraid and anxious lest your pain becomes so bad and persistent that your job and financial security are at risk. You may find that the effort of carrying on at work leaves you with little time, energy or enthusiasm for any enjoyment. It is quite common for people to manage reasonably well at work during the week, only to find that the weekend and holiday periods have to be used to recover. Migraine sufferers, particularly, become overwhelmed with their difficulties when the tension of working is relaxed. If you are in this situation then it is important that you take time to analyse it and decide whether there is anything you can do about it before you are overtaken by events and are forced to retire prematurely. In making your analysis the following suggestions may be helpful.

- Look at yourself, your personality and attitudes
  Consider:
- Are you a slave to duty? a perfectionist, demanding high standards of yourself and others?
- Are you always ready to indulge in self-blame?
- Are you over-critical of other people's faults?
- Are you dominated by ambition, by the need to achieve power, status and wealth?
- Do you often find yourself saying or thinking 'I should do this, I ought to do that, I should be able to achieve this?'
- Do you find it difficult to say NO and then be surprised to find that an already heavy workload gets even heavier?
- Do you carry on working through breaks?
- Do you find it difficult to schedule holidays, often failing to use up your holiday entitlement?
- Does anyone at work get you stirred up so that you find your pulse quickening, your chest tightening and your stomach muscles getting knotted?

118

- Do you find that you have to win arguments using energy to prove that you are right?
- Do you find that you are frequently standing on a point of principle?
- Are you driven by an anxious boss who implies that your achievements can always be bettered and is never satisfied even if the staff are working themselves to a standstill?
- Are you perhaps this boss?
- Is your work governed by unmanageable targets and threats of job loss if these are not achieved?
- Have you got caught up playing silly games where everyone feels the need to demonstrate keenness by arriving first each day and being the last one out at night, sometimes loaded down with work to finish at home?
- When driving, do you always drive to the limits of yourself and your vehicle feeling that you must pass everyone in front of you impatient with anyone who will impede your progress?
- Do you find yourself cutting others short in conversation so that you can say your piece?
- Do you grab a snack because you haven't the time for a proper lunch? And when you eat do you find yourself gulping your food down rather than chewing it thoroughly?

If you answer YES to a significant number of these questions and you have got pain, is it any wonder?

Isn't it about time that you began to make some changes before you lose control altogether? Your working life is a marathon, not a sprint! It is about survival, it is about enjoyment, family, friendships. It is about earning enough to meet your needs, leaving time and energy for fun and relaxation. Aim to get satisfaction from your work without damaging your health in the process.

Lucy was a teacher, married, with three teenage children. At 45 she was struggling at work in spite of severe neck and head pains which she had had for about four years. Investigations showed no physical cause.

When she was 40 she and her husband had taken out a large mortgage on a 'dream house'. Their joint incomes were stretched to meet the high repayments and to put their three children through college and university. This financial pressure coincided with the menopause and additional demands from a particularly troublesome class who tested her patience more than any other in her career. Her supportive, sympathetic headmaster retired and he was replaced by an over-demanding, ambitious 'whizz kid' keen to climb up the educational ladder on the backs of an overworked staff. He had the knack of provoking anxiety in others by innuendo and his demeanour was guaranteed to disturb a calm working atmosphere. The increased tension in the school transferred itself to an already unruly group of children. Each day on approaching her classroom, Lucy felt sick, her breathing quickened, her chest and tummy muscles tightened and this is how she stayed for most of the day. By the time she got home her shoulder and neck muscles were sore and uncomfortable.

You can appreciate Lucy's dilemma: she could give up work altogether, move to another school, find some way of continuing working in this unpleasant situation and probably get worse, OR she could take responsibility for improving her situation.

Lucy's problems were not amenable to a swift and easy solution but she was helped to regain some control by learning good relaxation and breathing techniques to use before setting out for school in the morning and at various points during the day. She was helped to develop more concern for her own well-being and to put limits on her desire to please and her readiness to accept all demands for extra work. She also took responsibility for planning her leisure time to include exercise and pleasurable activities with the family. This was only a beginning but the small improvements she felt made her examine her situation realistically and to plan much more positively with her husband for their future.

Getting back to work

For most people, work is very important. As well as a means of meeting financial needs it also brings opportunities to achieve status, power and prestige. We stress the importance of work so much that when we are denied the opportunity to work, for any reason at all, we experience a sense of loss and a feeling that we have been injured. Losing work because of illness which has an uncertain outcome, has an increased impact on the total personality of the individual adding to the loss of confidence, reduction in self-esteem to a point of possible depression and helplessness. As the prospect of getting back to work recedes as disablement increases, you begin to notice a deterioration in living standards and anxiety about getting back to work will increase.

All too often the illness or injury causing the pain may not be severe but the disability brought about by untreated or badly treated chronic pain reduces one's capacity to work. However, there is evidence from the treatment carried on at Walton Hospital, Liverpool and in Seattle, USA that people can be helped back into some kind of satisfactory working life.

Paradoxically, if you wish to get back to work you have to accept that a return to work is not the most important aim of your treatment. It may be, ultimately, but first things first. Your order of priority is: (1) increasing mobility (2) controlling pain (3) achieving a better quality and enjoyment of life (4) changing attitudes in order to redefine 'useful employment' (5) developing an ability to sustain effort for longer periods (6) assessing the need for training or retraining. I have covered the first of these three points in early chapters. We now need to look at points (4), (5) and (6).

It is important to take a broader view of work. It is understandable to feel a sense of panic about losing a job, particularly when you have to care for a family. There is a natural fear that your world will collapse if you are out of work. Your sole purpose in getting better is so that you can get back to your usual work as quickly as possible.

There may be many reasons why it is no longer possible to resume your normal employment after a long absence. There are obvious physical reasons but there may also be other legal or superannuation problems. Provided you reach a level of mobility and functioning which enables you to think once more about some form of employment, you may also need to think about the kind of employment which is suited to your present capacities. You may need help to think about re-training for something less exacting. You may even have to accept that the most important thing you can do is to find a way of becoming occupied in an absorbing task in order to give you a purpose in life and to prevent you becoming enslaved by your pain. Any activity which helps you to develop self-respect, self-esteem and which provides satisfaction can be defined as 'useful work', whether you are paid or not. Remember, being occupied in an absorbing task is one of the best distractions from pain.

No doubt at different times in your life things have happened to you which have been unpleasant and which at the time have left you devastated. No doubt as time has gone on you have been able to look back and see these events as experiences from which you have learned, possibly even making you stronger as a result. Try to look at your pain problem in the same way.

Before his illness, Bill's hobby had been ballroom dancing. As his mobility improved he began to look positively to the future. He was encouraged to think about using his dancing skills as the basis for a fuller recovery. He offered his services to a group of retired people as a ballroom dancing teacher, initially doing his work voluntarily and getting pleasure from the activity. It was not long before other groups called upon his services and, what is more, offered him a fee. This way he was able to supplement his income and at the same time he felt a sense of achievement and pride in his contribution to the pleasure of others.

Gordon and his wife had been given a large heated greenhouse by the family to mark their silver wedding anniversary. It had long been Gordon's wish to grow prize fuschias when he retired. Unfortunately, chronic pain had brought enforced premature retirement destroying all his hopes and ambitions for the future. However, as he began to get better, he started to think again about his plans for the greenhouse which had been standing idle and neglected for five years, a constant reminder of his incapacity and failed hopes. He became absorbed in reading specialist books on his favourite fuschias and gradually set about putting the greenhouse in order. Within two years Gordon's hobby was flourishing! and he was exploring the prospect of supplying hanging baskets to local garden centres.

These two examples demonstrate the possibilities arising from thinking differently about work and show that, with a positive approach, opportunities are available. My own personal experience of loss of a rewarding profession with all the attendant social and financial advantages was devastating and I felt that my usefulness as a bread-winner, a teacher, and therapist was over. In fact it was, for a period of six years. However, the very fact that I was a chronic pain sufferer became the foundation of an entirely new professional career in therapy, lecturing to patients and professionals involved in the field of pain management. Much of this work is carried out on a voluntary basis. Chronic pain has in fact enabled me to develop a completely new and satisfying way of life. Without it this book would never have been written.

Begin to look differently at your pain problem. As you improve, rather than seeing it as an obstacle, view it as a stepping-stone leading to different, and possibly better things.

When planning how to get back to work you *must* maximize your mobility and increase your stamina to the point where you can comfortably spend at least two hours at any job. This means building yourself up physically to cope with the demands of the task you are planning to do.

Again, the principle of gradual, progressive training, involving small increases in activity every day is paramount. Compare yourself to an athlete preparing for a marathon, building up slowly but surely. Be prepared to use to the full your new-found relaxation and breathing skills as frequently as possible during a working day and especially on your return home. Avoid being caught up in competition with the more physically able and accept your limitations without complaint.

Forget what you were once able to do. You can only depress yourself by comparing yourself to the person you were before your illness. Instead, take pride in stepping away from your 'disabled' status and always measure your progress by referring to the way you were at your lowest ebb. Remind yourself constantly that your own will, your own skills, your own efforts, are responsible for this improvement.

Not everyone will achieve a successful return to work even though physically they are capable of doing so.

Andy made a good recovery on the pain management course after being away from work for two years following a car accident. Before his accident he was a highly successful sales executive selling industrial machinery. But he overcame most of the physical weakness brought about by long inactivity, developed the capacity to relax and seemed to have recaptured his former positive approach to life. Andy's downfall had been his 'macho' attitude to his job and colleagues. He was not content to be a salesman – he wanted to be No. 1 salesman, the position he had held in his firm for a number of years.

Arrangements had been made for Andy to return to work gradually and his employer was fully prepared for him to take up the reins slowly. They hoped that, with his experience and background, he would eventually take up an administrative post in their busy sales office. This did not suit Andy's image of himself and he insisted on getting back on the road immediately, with a full workload, travelling 200 miles a day to have face-to-face contact with his customers. Reluctantly his employer agreed to this but by the end of six weeks Andy was burned out physically and emotionally. All the good work he had done with his rehabilitation had been forgotten. Fortunately, with appropriate counselling he was helped to make positive use of his failure, to accept his limitations, and to start all over again in a much more gradual manner, utilizing his energy to carry out his new tasks instead of wasting it on useless, destructive, competition.

10

Coping with Set-backs

Set-backs, relapses, or pain flare-ups are inevitable. For some people they can be destructive and become a major obstacle to ultimate rehabilitation, threatening to undo hard-earned progress. It is important to minimize the effects of set-back, and to arm against the likelihood of sustained relapse. Forewarned is fore-armed! It is important to take time to anticipate the ways in which they might occur and to devise ways to cope with them. Set-backs may easily happen as a result of trying to complete too large a task at any one time or setting a goal which is too ambitious for your stage of rehabilitation. The set-back is not a signal to give up altogether but to examine honestly the task set and to think of smaller, more manageable goals.

Malcolm, fired with enthusiasm for getting going again, jumped in with both feet and spent a Saturday doing a complete service on his car even to the extent of changing round all his wheels to spread out the wear on the tyres. He thoroughly enjoyed himself for many hours. However, he didn't return to the pain pro-gramme until Wednesday of the following week because he had been overwhelmed by pain for three days. He was full of remorse and was angry with the staff for encouraging him to get so involved. In analysing this with Malcolm it was apparent that he had completely ignored the advice to take manageable steps and build up slowly making sure of success at each stage of the exercise. He had reverted to behaving exactly as he did before he started with his pain problem. Fortunately, Malcolm was on the pain programme and he learned, with support, how to get back on the right track.

All too often people do get a set-back and begin to indulge in negative thinking saying to themselves: 'I'll never succeed, I'll never get any better. If I'm like this now what am I going to be like in the future?' It is so easy to indulge in self-defeating thoughts and self-condemnation, to label oneself as weak, inadequate, or worthless saying: 'Whatever I do I seem to get pain. What is wrong with me? What have I done to deserve this?' Learn to separate the past from the present and the present from the future. Regard each event in life as though it were the first time it has happened. It is important to get used to telling yourself this regularly. It is important, to recognize that if you have chronic pain you can easily become discouraged and slip into hopelessness, particularly at the beginning of treatment when you have had little experience of coping with set-backs. Begin to get into the habit of identifying progress and measuring your setbacks against the progress you have made. Make a habit of noting down in your diary information about the frequency, duration and intensity of pain. Progress does not occur dramatically but in small steps and it can often seem as though two steps forward are followed by three steps backwards. If you have data available as a result of ongoing self-monitoring, you can see for yourself that progress is in fact being made. Ask a friend or family member to remind you of what you were like before you started your recovery.

Often change is very subtle and it may be observed in only one area at a time, perhaps in a reduction of the frequency of pain, or the intensity or the duration, or it might only consist of a reduction in the amount of medication needed to control the pain. It is important to get used to taking note of the specific situations in which pain is experienced, taking note of your thoughts and feelings and of your reactions to it. Self-monitoring can help you identify factors that increase pain, such as anxiety or tension, and highlight the factors that reduce pain such as relaxation, listening to music, lovemaking, changing activities, planning treats, holidays, meeting friends, doing enjoyable hobbies.

It is important to accept that set-backs will take place and to develop a routine of thinking and behaving which will quickly get you back into equilibrium. First of all, accept the set-back as part of the normal experience and not as a catastrophe. Recognize it as a time to re-examine the progress you have made since you started your recovery and put the set-back into perspective. Accept that the flare-up may be a small price to pay for doing something which you have found enjoyable, exciting and rewarding.

My routine usually means that when I get a set-back it is a result of overdoing things. I do not always practise what I preach because I, too, like to get things done and don't like to miss out on anything! I take risks! And I pay the price from time to time. I have long since stopped condemning myself for being silly but recognize that I have the skill and the knowledge to help me through the difficult period. If necessary I will take myself through several periods of deep relaxation, reduce the demands made on me for a time and, as the pain subsides, go back to just enough exercise and activity to keep me ticking over until my energy returns – as it always does! Interestingly enough, I find that after a set-back I can often go on to a new higher level of achievement having taken stock mentally and physically and I can learn enough from the experience to devise new and better ways of coping. Set-backs can be positive!

The real demonstration of your ability to cope will be the day when you no longer deal with a set-back by

- staying in bed
- reaching for the medication
- rushing off to the doctor
- withdrawing from all activity
- falling back into bad habits and looking for sympathy.

Make a note of all the positive things that you can do to help yourself cope with a set-back.

Aids to maintaining normal functioning

Having worked hard over many years to regain control of my life, I have learned that the biggest danger during a set-back is to let slip away the pleasures and activities I have been enjoying. I have experienced the loss of a job, loss of status, loss of earning power, loss of hobbies, loss of the experience of performing on stage to a crowded auditorium. As I have learned to accept the reality of my condition and its limitations and have gained pleasure and pride from rebuilding my life and achieving new targets, I am determined that these gains will not be given up lightly. Anything which helps me to function will be considered. When I first lost my mobility as a result of pain I scorned the use of a wheelchair and crutches as symbols of giving up. I am now older and wiser and just as I appreciate the value of a car or bicycle to get me from A to B, from time to time I appreciate the use of a wheelchair which serves the same function. I am not dependent upon the wheelchair – it is my servant. I sometimes use it as a walking aid. It enables me to conserve energy and pace myself through a day. The energy saved can be spent on extending the time I can enjoy visits to art galleries or shopping centres. It also relieves the discomfort of standing around, shuffling along in a crowd, waiting at airports, etc., and removes from my partner the anxiety she feels for me in these situations. The result is that we both feel much more relaxed and our communication is not dominated by talk of my pain or my feelings of exhaustion.

My change in attitude resulted originally from a discussion I had with the physiotherapist at the local hospital after a severe set-back which affected my walking. She suggested that, as a temporary measure, elbow crutches should be used to take the weight off my spine, whilst at the same time making sure that I maintained as much mobility as possible and kept good posture. She also invited me to think about the positive value of using a wheelchair part of the time. I found this to be helpful during a holiday later on when I was able to spend much more time out of doors in a relaxed, comfortable seat. I found it a much better substitute for some of the very uncomfortable chairs in restaurants and, because of the folding facility of the chair, I was able to travel on trains and coaches and see much more of the countryside.

11

A New Partnership with your Doctor

Earlier chapters have focused on some of the changes you may need to consider and implement if you are to make progress in taking control of your life so that you are once more in a position to make choices. The ability to plan the future and to choose from a number of options seems to me to mark the difference between a healthy person and someone who is sick and dependent. Illness limits choice and creates dependence. It is a positive move for anyone suffering from illness to wish to eradicate the underlying problems. Unfortunately, illness of any kind also brings with it anxiety and panic so that when we approach our doctor we are not always emotionally in a state where we are able to choose between a number of options. We tend to rely on the doctor to put a name to our problem and to determine how it must be treated. We look outside ourselves for the answers, feel inhibited about asking too many questions and give our responsibility for our health up to the experts. This increases our dependence and we become passive recipients no longer in control of our own destiny.

You may have experienced a feeling of vagueness about medical consultations. This may not be because the doctor is vague and imprecise, but anxiety can get in the way of receiving clear-cut messages. You may hear what the doctor says but, because you are anxious about the outcome of the consultation, you may start putting your own interpretation on the message. A doctor, acting in good faith may, at the end of a series of tests and examinations, tell you that you have no life-threatening illness or disorder that needs surgery or hospitalization. Instead of hearing this reassuring message, it is possible to interpret this quite differently. You still have your pain, you are feeling angry, depressed and losing confidence. What you infer from his words is that there is nothing physically wrong with you and therefore he is implying that your pain is imaginery, or worse still, that you are neurotic or mentally ill. You may even feel that he is withholding bad news. This sort of misunderstanding can lead to an irrevocable breakdown in your relationship with your doctor.

It is possible for you to change your approach to medical consultations. It is easy to get into the habit of approaching your doctor complaining that you are no better – maybe even getting worse, looking more and more depressed and overwhelmed by your problem. This approach is likely to reinforce your doctor's feelings of inadequacy and to demonstrate his care for you he may be tempted to offer stronger drugs or more tests and investigations. So, try a different approach. Tell him you want to do something positive about your problem. If, as a result of reading this book, you recognize that you have chronic pain, then discuss with him the possibility of referral to a pain clinic as the first step in your rehabilitation. Seek his advice about increasing your mobility and strength and discuss a possible referral to a physiotherapist. Involve him in planning for your future well-being. Become more questioning about the reasons for investigations and what they entail.

If your doctor is proposing treatment with drugs or if he begins to write out a prescription without discussion, then be prepared with a line of questioning:

- What is the name of the drug?
- What is it for?
- It is specifically a pain-killer? Is it a tranquilizer? Is it a muscle-relaxant? Is it an anti-depressant?
- In what way will it help my pain?
- How often should I take it?
- How much should I take?
- How long will it be before I expect to feel an improvement?
- For how long do I need to take it?
- I am on other medication. How will this new one react with it?
- Is it safe to take alcohol or to drive?
- What side-effects might I expect to have in the short-term and in the long-term?
- If the tablets are withdrawn at a later date what will be the effects?

If you are already taking prescribed (or even over-the-counter) medication, begin to ask yourself whether these tablets really have a beneficial effect on your pain or are they acting in such a way that you feel less pain because they are numbing your senses generally, making you feel drowsy or detached from what is going on around you. Ask yourself whether you have just got into the habit of taking tablets – 'just in case'. Are you taking stronger and more frequent doses to get the same relief from your pain? Do you fall into the category of many people who just ring their doctor and ask for a repeat prescription without taking the initiative and asking the doctor to review what the tablets are in fact achieving.

If you are unhappy about the effects of your medication and you are keen to seek relief in other ways, then ask your GP about reducing the medication you are taking. *Do not* suddenly stop taking any prescribed medication which you have been taking for a long time as the effects of sudden withdrawal may be unpleasant. Your doctor will know how to reduce your dosage safely and systematically making sure that one type of medication only is reduced at a time.

12
And . . . Finally!

I have avoided going into great detail about other professional services which are available to help the pain sufferer. Be warned, though, there are enormous commercial interests supplying services and products to alleviate or 'cure' pain. Advertising is a powerful tool which can create anxieties and raise hopes. As a result you could spend a fortune trying to find a cure which might not be there. You will not be in a position to spend money on a large scale for a long period – perhaps for life, so think first of simple remedies to ease your discomfort.

The old-fashioned hot water bottle is just as effective as any other means of providing localized warmth. Heat, whatever its source, is comforting and promotes better circulation around an injured or sore part of the body. A warm bath or shower may be sufficient to bring relief or play its part in promoting your relaxation. Embrocations, balms, sprays, hot or cold are also very useful and might be obtainable on prescription. If a cold spray is not available, a bag of frozen peas or an ice-pack wrapped in a cloth will act just as well. Experiment with the application of heat and with cold and see which suits you best. I find that heat applied when I can feel pain coming on can prevent it growing to intolerable levels. Warmth during relaxation periods can be very helpful.

If you can learn to recognize the signs of the onset of pain and take action straight away instead of pressing on and increasing your tension you will find you can cope with it much more easily. For example, at the first sign, change your position or stop the activity you are doing and do something else. Alternatively, if necessary, take a mild pain-killer, such as aspirin or paracetamol, one which suits you, and relax completely, allowing your body to take care of the pain in its own way.

We have already talked about the virtues of gentle massage and rubbing and finding ways to distract yourself from your pain. There are some people whose arms or legs itch or burn intolerably, technically known as causalgia and this can be most distressing. I have found relief by the application of very cold wet compresses which allow me sufficient respite to relax or get off to sleep.

You might wish from time to time to supplement your own resources which are the *most important* by seeking help from a variety of professionals, for example, acupuncturists, osteopaths, chiropractors, hypnotherapists and homeopaths. As with your GP or other medical consultants you have been to, you must not allow them to take complete responsibility for your health and well-being. They can offer specific treatments to bolster your own resources but they are not miracle workers.

Self-help groups

Self-help groups are being set up throughout the country. This is a valuable step forward and reflects the growing realization that people are very effective in helping each other through their own experience. One can only applaud those people who, in spite of their own problems, find the time and energy to take responsibility for organizing and running these groups.

Unfortunately, in the case of pain management, self-help groups often exist to fill the void rather than a gap in provision. There seems to come a point where national resources cease to be allocated in order to reactivate and instead money is spent on making provisions for the disabled. Now do not misunderstand, there *must* be provision for people with disability but it often seems to patients who are trying their best to get back to a normal lifestyle that it is better to give up, become completely disabled, then enjoy the services which are available. The cost of getting one person back to normal functioning is negligible when compared with the cost of maintaining that same person in a disabled status throughout his whole life.

You will recall that at the start of this book I referred to the high percentage of the ageing population suffering disability from chronic pain. These people deserve to be living with the highest possible quality of life that can be obtained through their own, or society's efforts. Are they to be fobbed off with drugs which depress the spirit, and kept quiet within the confines of their homes or sheltered accommodation rather than being helped and encouraged through good pain management techniques to live their lives as they wish –and to the full?

Most communities have well-furnished, warm and comfortable

health centres, sports and leisure centres, and swimming complexes. I would like to see these used fully in an organized way to promote good health and to prevent disability among chronic pain sufferers. If you accept that 10% of the population has chronic pain it means that over 5 million people individually make use of the health centres, absorbing millions of pounds worth of prescribed drugs, following each other round from consultant to consultant, hospital to hospital and possibly getting nowhere. A good pain management programme which focuses on all aspects of the problem, physical, emotional, and social, would do much to reduce the load on the doctors' surgeries and the hospitals and would provide a positive service to a significant number of the population who feel they are forgotten. It is a sad indictment on our well-resourced National Health Service that skilled professional workers are not brought together more frequently under one roof to deal with groups of patients at one time over an intensive three- or four-week period. Instead, more often than not, each doctor, each physiotherapist, each occupational- and psychotherapist in turn deals individually with patients who have often waited weeks or even months for an appointment. It is this system which can be instrumental in creating intractable problems. What a waste of resources!

If this state of affairs continues then self-help groups may continue to proliferate unsupported, without the necessary knowledge and skills. They may provide a useful social outlet or act as pressure groups but there is a possibility that because they are not part of The System and are given no professional guidance, they will do little or nothing to reactivate people but merely support them in their disability.

This book has set out primarily to help you to understand and highlight the way in which your own physical and mental resources might be enhanced so that you develop an increased ability to take control of your pain – and, of course, of your life. I have attempted to demonstrate the ways in which it is possible to become more active, more mobile and more involved so that you can take a fuller part in the life of your family, friends and workmates. It is my hope that it has provided some help and comfort to people who feel neglected. I have tried to demonstrate that the knowledge and skills necessary to treat chronic pain are there and to show how professionals working together on pain management can help people who have been written off to achieve comfortable and satisfactory lives. A book is a poor substitute for an effective pain management programme but hopefully you will have been inspired to take steps to work on your own rehabilitation. Ultimately, the major task of pain management belongs to YOU!

This is the point at which the first edition of my book ended. Since then there have been many significant changes which need to be placed on record. Pain is now on the agenda at all levels. In 1993 the Department of Health accepted that chronic pain is a condition which needs treatment in its own right and, as a result, there have been surveys of resources and provision undertaken in various parts of the country. These have led to the publication of hospital guidelines for the treatment of pain. At the moment, hospital provision for pain relief is not consistent throughout the country. There will need to be a great deal of research to assess the real demand for resources before anyone can set up programmes adequate to meet the needs. One vital step has been taken. It is now possible for GPs to refer patients directly to a pain clinic, whereas, previously, referrals could only be made via a hospital consultant. Many hospitals are now considering what is an appropriate budget for staffing clinics and providing medication and equipment. A number of hospital districts are now providing pain management courses to supplement the work of their pain clinic, and others are exploring the possibility of making this kind of provision. If you are not aware of this provision in your area, then keep on asking your GP about these facilities. If there are none in your area, then you can request that your GP provides the funds to enable you to get this treatment outside your area. Information about facilities can be obtained from one of the pain charities who provide telephone helplines and information services. Addresses and telephone numbers are given at the end of the book. It is good to see that these charities are now being supported fully by the medical profession, the Department of Health, by industry and local authorities.

After the publication of the first edition of this book, I received many letters from people who have been encouraged to take their first steps on the way to recovery, regaining confidence and having more control over their lives. I also received many requests for help and advice about setting up and running community-based programmes. I have long believed that no matter how generous the treatment for chronic pain might be within a hospital setting, people with chronic pain need to have the opportunity for learning and continuous support within the community. Very few of the millions who have the problem will actually be referred to a hospital for treatment and therefore something else is needed. In the last three years I have been working towards developing methods of working which are appropriate to self-help groups operating within the community, with members being responsible for running them. The methods devised are focused on education and learning rather than treatment. Effective learning is in itself therapeutic insofar as it helps people to work towards complete reliance on their own inner resources to cope with the problem of pain.

In sharing ways in which they cope (or didn't cope), each may learn something which may be of value and support as they use their group membership as a platform, to enable them to learn new skills and make changes. The group can provide a safe environment where an appropriate level of trust can develop, and as people interact more easily with each other they may recognize they are not as different, isolated or incompetent as they thought. A group brings together people who possess specialist knowledge and experience not commonly available to others. The professionals' knowledge of chronic pain and its treatment may be profound, but this knowledge is of a different quality from that of people who actually live with the problem. People in chronic pain share the experience of having a problem which appears to be intractable in spite of the best efforts of the medical profession. They share feelings of abandonment, anger and even rage, loss, frustration, depression and helplessness; feelings which add considerably to the burden of pain. It is most important for people with pain to learn in normal community surroundings: schools, community centres leisure centres, adult education centres, church groups – in fact anywhere which takes the focus off them as 'sick' people.

Using this educational approach, 'pilot' courses have been established, under the sponsorship of Pain Association Scotland, who have a long-standing track record in providing a wide range of support for people with pain throughout the community. The aims of these groups have been clearly stated as:

1. Reactivation and maintenance of mobility.
2. Relief of tension and development of relaxation.
3. Involvement in purposeful activity with others leading to changes in attitudes and behaviour.
4. The encouragement of people with pain to run their own self-help pain management programme.

Learning in the group situation carries a great deal of conviction and, in particular, there are two major advantages:

1. The recognition that others have coped with similar problems.
2. The message seems to have more credibility and learning is more rapid when conveyed by a group of people who have firsthand experience.

Feedback from those who took part was tremendously encouraging and the results exceeded expectations. The course material used has now been put together in the form of a training manual which consists of information about planning for group work, recruiting and communicating with members, group management and leadership, sample timetables, scripts, leaders' notes, tapes and printed handouts. The manual is designed for use by groups, especially by people with pain working independently, or in conjunction with professional help. The full training manual can be purchased from Pain Association Scotland.

As you begin to improve, remember that it is always useful to have someone who understands your situation to talk to during dangerous set-back periods. If you do not have access to group support or you are physically isolated from other people with pain, then ask one of the Pain Charities to put you in touch with one of their members, by telephone if necessary. It is useful to belong to a network of people who share your problems and are working in a positive way to cope with their pain. It is important to have someone to encourage you to carry on with learning pain management techniques; to help you examine your situation honestly; and to tell you to 'pull your finger out' occasionally! It is *not* helpful to have someone around who encourages you to sit back and permanently adopt the role of an invalid.

You make your own luck! It is possible to achieve more with your life if you have chronic pain than many so-called perfectly healthy people. By taking small steps and following all the things you have learned from this book, you can get more enjoyment and more satisfaction out of every day than most people. Try to look upon your pain and the skills you are learning as providing an opportunity to move forward.

You only have one life, so live it to the full – enjoy it!

Useful Addresses

Physiotherapy. The Chartered Society of Physiotherapy, 14 Bedford Row, London WC1R 4ED. Tel. 020–7242–1941

Osteopathy. The General Council and Register of Osteopaths, 56 London Street, Reading, Berks RG1 4SQ. Tel. 0118 957 6585

Chiropractic. The British Chiropractic Association, Blagrave House, 17 Blagrave Street, Reading, Berks RG1 1QB. Tel. 0118 950 5950

Acupuncture. The Acupuncture Association and Register, 34 Alderney Street, London SW1V 4EU. Tel. 020–7834–1012

General Information and specific details about Qualified Hypnotherapists: The Institute for Complementary Medicine, PO Box 194, London SE16 1QZ. Tel. 020–7237–5165

Backcare, The Old Office Block, 16 Elmtree Road, Teddington, Middlesex TW11 8ST. Tel. 020–8977–5474

The British Homeopathic Association, 27A Devonshire Street, London W1N 1RG

The Society of Homeopaths, 4a Artizan Road, Northampton NN1 4HU. Tel. 01604 621400

Self-Help Groups: Pain Association Scotland, Cramond House, Kirk Cramond, Cramond Glebe Road, Edinburgh EH4 6NS. Tel. 0131–312–7955 (office and helpline – for people with chronic pain, including cancer pain)

Pain Concern (UK), PO Box 318, Canterbury Kent CT4 5DP. Telephone helpline 01227 264677 (Mon-Fri 10am to 4pm)

Arthritis Care, 18 Stephenson Way, London NW1 2HD. Tel. 020–7916–1500; Helpline 0800 289170, 12 noon to 4pm

The National Federation of Spiritual Healers, Old Manor Farm Studio, Church Street, Sunbury-on-Thames, Middx TW16 6RG. Tel. 01932 783164

Short Residential Courses: Information about these can be obtained from National Institute of Adult Continuing Education (NIACE) 19B De Montfort Street, Leicester LE1 7GE. Tel. 0116 2551451

Henleys Medical Supplies Ltd., Brownfields, Welwyn Garden City, Herts AL7 1AN. Tel. 01707 333164 who kindly supplied the author with one of their Biotens TU1000 machines for trial purposes.

The Biofeedback Machine for home use can be obtained through any Tandy dealer.

Relaxation tapes

Tapes prepared by the author, supplementary to this book can be purchased at a nominal charge from Pain Association Scotland, Cramond House, Kirk Cramond, Cramond Glebe Road, Edinburgh EH4 6NS.

Self-help manual

A Community-Based Pain Management Programme by Neville Shone is published by Pain Assocation Scotland and can be purchased from the above address.

Index